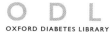

O D L
OXFORD DIABETES LIBRARY

Heart Disease and Diabetes

D1275003

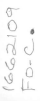

▶ Except where otherwise stated, drug doses and recommendations are for the non-pregnant adult who is not breast-feeding.

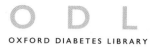

OXFORD DIABETES LIBRARY

Heart Disease and Diabetes

Edited by

Dr Miles Fisher

Consultant Physician,
Glasgow Royal Infirmary, UK

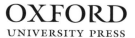

OXFORD
UNIVERSITY PRESS

OXFORD
UNIVERSITY PRESS

Great Clarendon Street, Oxford OX2 6DP

Oxford University Press is a department of the University of Oxford.
It furthers the University's objective of excellence in research, scholarship,
and education by publishing worldwide in

Oxford New York

Auckland Cape Town Dar es Salaam Hong Kong Karachi
Kuala Lumpur Madrid Melbourne Mexico City Nairobi
New Delhi Shanghai Taipei Toronto

With offices in

Argentina Austria Brazil Chile Czech Republic France Greece
Guatemala Hungary Italy Japan Poland Portugal Singapore
South Korea Switzerland Thailand Turkey Ukraine Vietnam

Oxford is a registered trade mark of Oxford University Press
in the UK and in certain other countries

Published in the United States
by Oxford University Press Inc., New York

© Oxford University Press, 2008

British Library Cataloguing in Publication Data

Data available

Library of Congress Cataloging in Publication Data

Data available

Typeset by Newgen Imaging Systems (P) Ltd., Chennai, India
Printed in Great Britain
on acid-free paper by
Ashford Colour Press Ltd., Gosport, Hampshire

ISBN 978–0–19–954372–4

10 9 8 7 6 5 4 3 2 1

Contents

Preface

It is interesting to reflect on how the approach to heart disease in people with diabetes has changed in the last fourteen years. Previously heart disease in people with diabetes was thought to be irreversible, and the clinical approach was pessimistic. The research approach was little better, and people with diabetes were often excluded from large cardiovascular trials in case their vascular disease obscured possible benefits in non-diabetic subjects.

Slowly evidence emerged from lipid, blood pressure, glycaemic, and other cardiovascular studies that people with diabetes did indeed respond to pharmacological and physical interventions, that the relative response was often similar to that in non-diabetic people, but as the event rate was much higher a greater reduction in absolute risk was obtained.

Diabetes is now seen as a cardiovascular disease equivalent, but it remains disappointing that measures to improve glycaemic control have relatively minor effects on reducing cardiovascular events compared to lipid and blood pressure interventions. It is also disappointing that certain sub-groups of diabetic patients, e.g. those with diabetic nephropathy or autonomic neuropathy, have few evidence-based therapies to reduce cardiovascular risk and the risk of dying.

This book is a concise and practical guide to reducing cardiovascular risk and in particular heart disease in people with diabetes. It should be of interest to GPs and practice nurses, hospital specialists and specialist nurses in diabetes and cardiology, and also contains something of interest for renal physicians and stroke doctors.

I am extremely grateful to the other authors for their contributions to this book. Stephen Wheatcroft and his cardiology colleagues from Leeds have provided the more cardiological chapters. My diabetes work colleague Dr Ken Paterson, now the chair of the Scottish Medicines Consortium, along with clinical pharmacology colleagues, has produced a very useful, and for a clinician understandable, guide to the health economic aspects of treating cardiovascular disease in diabetes. I thank them all for their contributions.

Finally, I wish to thank my wife Margaret and son Marc, who again have had to suffer evenings and weekends where I have been present in the household but absent from the family, while doing battle with a laptop computer. I hope that they, and you the reader, agree that this has been time well spent.

Miles Fisher, June 2008.

Contributors

Ailsa Brown
Principal Health Economist,
Scottish Medicines Consortium,
Glasgow, UK

Joyce Craig
Lead Health Economist,
NHS Quality Improvement
Scotland,
Glasgow, UK

Dr Miles Fisher
Consultant Physician,
Glasgow Royal Infirmary,
Glasgow, UK

**Dr Matthew Kahn BSc,
MRCP**
Clinical Research Fellow,
Division of Cardiovascular and
Diabetes Research,
Leeds Institute of Genetics,
Health and Therapeutics,
LIGHT Laboratories,
University of Leeds,
Leeds, UK

Dr Ken Paterson
Consultant Physician,
Glasgow Royal Infirmary,
Glasgow, UK

Dr Adil Rajwani BSc, MRCP
Clinical Research Fellow,
Division of Cardiovascular and
Diabetes Research,
Leeds Institute of Genetics,
Health and Therapeutics,
LIGHT Laboratories,
University of Leeds,
Leeds, UK

**Dr Stephen Wheatcroft
BSc, PhD, MRCP**
British Heart Foundation
Intermediate Clinical Research
Fellow/Consultant Cardiologist,
Division of Cardiovascular and
Diabetes Research,
Leeds Institute of Genetics,
Health and Therapeutics,
LIGHT Laboratories,
University of Leeds, Leeds, UK

Contents

Abbreviations

ABPM	ambulatory blood pressure monitoring
ACE	angiotensin-converting enzyme
AGE	advanced glycation end products
ADVANCE	Action in Diabetes and Vascular disease: preterAx and diamicroN-MR Controlled Evaluation
ALLHAT	Antihypertensive and Lipid-Lowering treatment to prevent Heart Attack Trial
ARAs	Angiotensin-II receptor antagonists
ARTS	Arterial Revascularization Therapies Study
ASCOT	Anglo-Scandinavian Cardiac Outcomes Trial
AT_1	angiotensin 1
ATP	Adult Treatment Panel
AWESOME	Angina With Extremely Serious Operative Mortality Evaluation
BARI	Bypass Angioplasty Revascularization Investigation
BNP	brain natriuretic peptide
CABG	coronary artery bypass graft
CAN	cardiovascular autonomic neuropathy
CAPRIE	Clopidogrel versus Aspirin in Patients at Risk of Ischaemic Events
CARDIA	Coronary Artery Revascularisation in DIAbetes
CARDS	Collaborative AtoRvastatin Diabetes Study
CARE	Cholesterol and Recurrent Events
CHD	coronary heart disease
CHF	chronic heart failure
CIMT	carotid intima-media thickness
CORE	Centre for Outcomes Research
CRP	C-reactive protein
CTT	Cholesterol Treatment Trialists
CURE	Clopidogrel in Unstable angina to Reduce Recurrent Events
CVD	cardiovascular disease
DCCT	Diabetes Control and Complications Trial
DETAIL	Diabetics Exposed to Telmisartan and Enalapril

DIABHYCAR	Diabetes, Hypertension, cardiovascular events, and Ramipril
DM	diabetes mellitus
DPP	Diabetes Prevention Program
DPP-4	dipeptidyl pepitidase-4
DPS	Diabetes Prevention Study
DREAM	Diabetes Reduction Assessment with ramipril and rosiglitazone Medication
ECG	electrocardiography
ED	erectile dysfunction
EDIC	Epidemiology of Diabetes Interventions and Complications
ESRD	end-stage renal disease
ET-1	endothelin
FIELD	Fenofibrate Intervention and Event Lowering in Diabetes
FREEDOM	Future REvascularisation Evaluation in patients with Diabetes mellitus: Optimal Management
GIP	glucose-dependent insulinotropic peptide
GIST-UK	The UK Glucose Insulin in Stroke Trial
GLP-1	Glucagon-like peptide 1
HDL	High-density Lipoprotein
HOPE	Heart Outcomes Prevention Evaluation
HOT	Hypertension Optimal Treatment
HPS	Heart Protection Study
HR	high risk
ICDs	implantable cardiac defibrillators
ICER	incremental cost-effectiveness ratio
IDNT	Irbesartan Diabetic Nephropathy Trial
IFG	impaired fasting glucose
IGT	impaired glucose tolerance
IL-6	interleukin-6
IRMA-2	Irbesartan in Patients with Type 2 Diabetes and Microalbuminuria Study
LDL	low-density Lipoprotein
LIFE	Losartan Intervention For Endpoint reduction in hypertension

LIPID	Long-Term Intervention with Pravastatin in Ischaemic Disease
LVSD	left ventricular systolic dysfunction
MARVAL	Microalbuminuria Reduction with Valsartan
MI	myocardial infarction
MIBG	meta-iodobenzylguanidine
MICRO-HOPE	Microalbuminuria, Cardiovascular and Renal Outcomes in the Heart Outcomes Prevention Evaluation
NICE	National Institute for Health and Clinical Excellence
NO	nitric oxide
NOD	new-onset diabetes
NYHA	New York Heart Association
OGTT	oral glucose tolerance test
PAD	peripheral arterial disease
PCI	percutaneous coronary intervention
PDE5	phosphodiesterase type-5
PPAR gamma	peroxisome-proliferator-activated receptor gamma
PPV	Positive prediction value
PROactive	PROspective pioglitAzone Clinical Trial In macro Vascular Events
PROGRESS	Perindopril Protection against Recurrent Stroke Study
PROVE-IT TIMI 22	Pravastatin or Atorvastatin Evaluation and Infection Therapy-Thrombolysis in Myocardial Infraction 22
PTCA	Percutaneous Transluminal Coronary Angioplasty
QALY	Quality Adjusted Life Year
REACH	Reduction of Atherothrombosis for Continued Health
RECORD	Rosiglitazone Evaluated for Cardiac Outcomes and Regulation of glycaemia in Diabetes
SCOUT	Sibutramine Cardiovascular Outcomes Trial
SHEP	Systolic Hypertension in the Elderly Program
4S	The Scandinavian Simvastatin Survival Study
SMC	Scottish Medicines Consortium
SOS	stents or surgery

SPARCL	Stroke Prevention by Aggressive Reduction in Cholesterol Levels
STOP-NIDDM	Study to Prevent Non-Insulin-Dependent Diabetes Mellitus
Syst-Eur	Systolic hypertension-Europe
TIAs	transient ischaemic attacks
TNT	Treatment to New Targets
TZD	thiazolidinedione
UKPDS	United Kingdom Prospective Diabetes Study
VLDLs	very low density lipoproteins
WOSCOPS	The West of Scotland Coronary Prevention Study
XENDOS	XENical in the prevention of Diabetes in Obese Subjects

Chapter 1

Introduction, epidemiology, and cardiovascular risk factors

Miles Fisher

Diabetes is a state of premature cardiovascular death which is associated with chronic hyperglycaemia and may also be associated with blindness and renal failure.

Miles Fisher, British Diabetic Association meeting Dublin 1996.

> ### Key points
>
> - Cardiovascular disease is a common cause of morbidity and mortality in people with type 2 diabetes. Several guidelines define diabetes as a coronary heart disease equivalent, requiring multiple cardiovascular risk factor reduction.
> - In addition to diabetes the World Health Organisation (WHO) has defined two pre-diabetic states of impaired glucose tolerance and impaired fasting glucose. Subjects with pre-diabetes have an increased risk of cardiovascular disease, and of progression to diabetes.
> - The presence of the metabolic syndrome (abdominal obesity, diabetes or pre-diabetes, raised blood pressure, and dyslipidaemia) predicts subsequent development of diabetes and vascular disease, but is not at present a separate target for intervention.
> - The relative risk of cardiovascular disease is greatly increased in people with type 1 diabetes, but the absolute risk is not particularly high. Components of the metabolic syndrome predict cardiovascular risk in type 1 diabetes.

1.1 **Introduction**

When I suggested the above re-definition of diabetes, which was prior to the publication of the results of the United Kingdom Prospective Diabetes Study (UKPDS), only the treatment of hypercholesterolaemia and hypertension, plus the use of antiplatelet drugs in certain high-risk patients, were of proven benefit in reducing cardiovascular events in people with diabetes. The purpose of the re-definition was to awaken healthcare professionals caring for people with diabetes to the fact that clinical management needed to embrace the prevention, detection, and treatment of macrovascular disease in addition to microvascular disease.

1.2 **Epidemiology**

The Framingham study was one of the first to quantify the increased risk of cardiovascular morbidity and mortality in people with diabetes, and showed that there was an excess of cardiovascular disease in people with diabetes (predominantly type 2 diabetes) compared to that in non-diabetic people. This could not be fully explained by conventional cardiovascular risk factors of blood pressure, cholesterol, smoking, or obesity. Excesses were demonstrated in coronary heart disease, congestive cardiac failure, strokes, peripheral vascular disease, and cardiovascular deaths (Table 1.1). In particular, an excess cardiovascular morbidity and mortality was seen in women with diabetes, and the rates of vascular disease in diabetic women approached the rates of vascular disease in men with diabetes.

In a study based on a database from Finland it was shown that people with type 2 diabetes, who had no known cardiac disease, had the same incidence of myocardial infarction and cardiovascular death on 7-year follow-up as people without diabetes who had sustained a myocardial infarction. Similar results were obtained on 18-year follow-up (Figure 1.1). Others have challenged the suggestion that diabetes is a

Table 1.1 Increased risk of cardiovascular disease in diabetic subjects compared to non-diabetic subjects in the Framingham study		
	Relative risk men	**Relative risk women**
Coronary heart disease	2	3
Stroke	2	4
Peripheral arterial disease	4	6
Congestive heart failure	2	5
Any cardiovascular disease	2	3
Cardiovascular death	2	5

true coronary heart disease equivalent, pointing out that while the event rate in people with diabetes who are completely free of vascular disease at baseline is increased compared to that in non-diabetic subjects, the event rate is not as high as in survivors of myocardial infarction (Figure 1.2). It is worth noting that in all studies the event rate is greatly increased in diabetic patients who have already had a previous myocardial infarction (Figure 1.1).

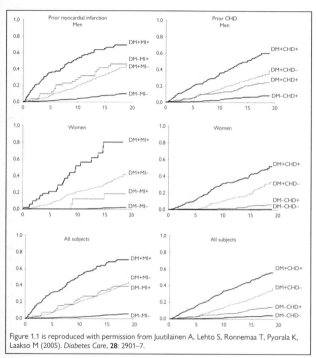

Figure 1.1 is reproduced with permission from Juutilainen A, Lehto S, Ronnemaa T, Pyorala K, Laakso M (2005). *Diabetes Care*, **28**: 2901–7.

Figure 1.1 Coronary heart disease mortality during an 18-year follow-up according to the presence of diabetes (DM), prior myocardial infarction (MI) and prior coronary heart disease (CHD) comprising ECG changes, angina, or prior myocardial infarction.

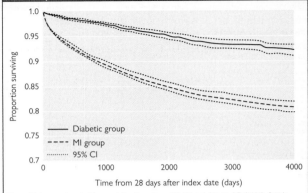

Figure 1.2 Survival curve for cardiovascular death in patients with newly diagnosed type 2 diabetes and patients who just had a myocardial infarction (MI)

Figure 1.2 is reproduced with permission from Evans JM, Wang J, Morris AD (2002). *British Medical Journal*, **324**: 939–42.

1.2.1 Risk factors for coronary heart disease in diabetes

The UKPDS was a large randomized trial of intensive versus conventional treatment of blood glucose in patients with recently diagnosed type 2 diabetes. A large amount of epidemiological data has been obtained from the study. In the UKPDS at baseline the traditional risk markers of hypertension, dyslipidaemia, and smoking, as well as HbA1c were independent risk factors for subsequent coronary events, indicating a potential for risk factor intervention in people with type 2 diabetes (Table 1.2). The importance of HbA1c as a risk factor is that it indicated that it was not just the presence of diabetes but the degree of hyperglycaemia as measured by HbA1c that was important. Variation in fasting blood glucose and HbA1c within the normal range has been shown to predict cardiovascular risk within the non-diabetic population. In this way, glycaemia as a risk factor is similar to cholesterol and blood pressure.

More recently several novel risk markers have been shown to predict cardiovascular risk in diabetes, including endothelial dysfunction, microalbuminuria and reduced glomerular filtration rate, fibrinogen and other markers of haemostasis, and C-reactive protein (CRP) and other markers of inflammation.

Table 1.2 Risk factors for coronary heart disease and myocardial infarction in the UKPDS (UKPDS 23, Turner et al. 1998)		
Coronary artery disease	Fatal or non-fatal myocardial infarction	Fatal myocardial infarction
Raised LDL cholesterol	Raised LDL cholesterol	Diastolic blood pressure
Low HDL cholesterol	Diastolic blood pressure	Raised LDL cholesterol
HbA1c	Smoking	HbA1c
Systolic blood pressure	Low HDL cholesterol	
Smoking	HbA1c	

Reproduced with permission from Turner RC, Millns H, Neil HAW, Stratton IM, Manley SE, Matthews DR, Holman RR, (1998). Risk factors for coronary artery disease in non-insulin dependent diabetes mellitus: United Kingdom Prospective Diabetes Study (UK PDS:23). *British Medical Journal*, **316**: 823–8.

1.2.2 Risk estimation

Cardiovascular risk tables have been used to estimate risk in asymptomatic individuals, and to make decisions on possible treatment of dyslipidaemia or hypertension. Many risk tables are based on data obtained from Framingham. This method of risk estimation is much less accurate in diabetic subjects for several reasons:

- There were few subjects with diabetes in the Framingham cohort that was used to derive the Framingham equation.
- The typical dyslipidaemia of diabetes comprises a relatively normal total cholesterol or LDL cholesterol, but with a higher concentration of the more atherogenic small, dense LDL (Chapter 3).
- Patients were not characterized according to type of diabetes, and most were presumed to have type 2 diabetes in this age group, so data are lacking for patients with type 1 diabetes.
- Framingham studied a largely white population, so does not take account of ethnicity. It has been shown that many diabetic ethnic minority groups, such as South Asians in the United Kingdom, are at a higher risk than the majority population.
- It does not take account of microalbuminuria or novel risk markers.

A possible approach to this problem is to use a method of estimating risk that is unique for diabetes, such as the UKPDS risk engine. Another approach is to accept that people with diabetes have a coronary risk equivalent to existing CHD in non-diabetic subjects and to treat accordingly. This approach was first adopted in the Adult Treatment Panel (ATP) III guidelines in the United States, and more recently by the revised Joint British Society Guidelines.

1.3 **Pre-diabetes**

The current WHO diagnostic criteria for the diagnosis of diabetes are based on the subsequent development of microvascular complications, particularly retinopathy, and not macrovascular complications. Two pre-diabetic states are also described—impaired glucose tolerance and impaired fasting glucose (Table 1.3). Both of these predict the subsequent development of diabetes, and are associated with an increased risk of cardiovascular disease. Impaired glucose tolerance (IGT) is a better predictor of cardiovascular disease than impaired fasting glucose (IFG), supporting the suggestion that postprandial glucose excursions may be a more important contributor to vascular events than fasting glucose.

The progression from pre-diabetes to diabetes can be delayed by changes in lifestyle and pharmacological therapy, but so far only acarbose has been shown to reduce cardiovascular events (Table 1.4).

Table 1.3 Diagnostic criteria for diabetes, impaired glucose tolerance, and impaired fasting glucose

Diabetes mellitus	Impaired glucose tolerance	Impaired fasting glucose
Random plasma glucose ≥ 11.1mmol/L *Or* Fasting plasma glucose ≥ 7.0mmol/L *Or* 2 hour plasma glucose ≥ 11.1mmol/L on oral glucose tolerance test (OGTT)	Fasting plasma glucose <7.0mmol/L *And* 2-hour plasma glucose 7.8–11.0mmol/L on OGTT	Fasting plasma glucose 6.0–6.9mmol/L (WHO criteria) *Or* Fasting plasma glucose 5.6–6.9 (ADA criteria)

Table 1.4 Effects of interventions to reduce the progression to diabetes on cardiovascular risk markers or cardiovascular events

Intervention	Effect on cardiovascular risk
Lifestyle change	Reduced weight, blood pressure, triglycerides, increased HDL cholesterol, improved fibrinolysis
Metformin	Reduced weight
Acarbose	Reduced major cardiovascular events and new hypertension
Orlistat	Reduced blood pressure, total and LDL cholesterol
Rosiglitazone	Increased weight, insignificant increase in cardiovascular events

1.3.1 **Lifestyle measures in pre-diabetes**

The effects of changes in diet and increased physical activity on the progression to diabetes were examined in the Finnish Diabetes Prevention Study (DPS) and the American Diabetes Prevention Program (DPP). In the DPP, lifestyle change was more effective than metformin in reducing the progression to diabetes. Changes in cardiovascular risk factors are shown in Table 1.4. Observational follow-up of the DPP is being performed to see if these changes in cardiovascular risk factors lead to a reduction in cardiovascular events.

1.3.2 **Acarbose in pre-diabetes**

In the Study to Prevent Non-Insulin-Dependent Diabetes Mellitus (STOP-NIDDM) trial acarbose delayed the progression to diabetes in patients with IGT. In a post hoc analysis, patients in the acarbose group had a significant reduction in a cardiovascular composite outcome that included CHD, cardiovascular death, congestive cardiac failure, strokes, and peripheral vascular disease (Figure 1.3). There was also a significant reduction in the development of hypertension.

1.3.3 **Orlistat in pre-diabetes**

In the XENical in the prevention of Diabetes in Obese Subjects (XENDOS) study, orlistat delayed the progression to diabetes, particularly in subjects with IGT. Weight was reduced with orlistat, and there were greater reductions in systolic and diastolic blood pressure and total and LDL cholesterol. HbA1c and cardiovascular events were not reported.

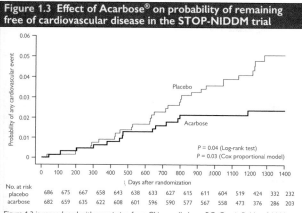

Figure 1.3 Effect of Acarbose® on probability of remaining free of cardiovascular disease in the STOP-NIDDM trial

$P = 0.04$ (Log-rank test)
$P = 0.03$ (Cox proportional model)

No. at risk														
placebo	686	675	667	658	643	638	633	627	615	611	604	519	424	332	232
acarbose	682	659	635	622	608	601	596	590	577	567	558	473	376	286	203

Figure 1.3 is reproduced with permission from Chiasson JL, Josse RG, Gomis R, Hanefeld M, Karasik A, Laakso M. For the STOP-NIDDM Trial Research Group (2003). *Journal of American Medical Association*, **290**: 486–94.

1.3.4 **Glitazones in pre-diabetes**

One arm of the DPP was the use of troglitazone, but this arm was discontinued because of hepatic toxicity, including a subject in DPP who died from liver failure. In the Diabetes Reduction Assessment with ramipril and rosiglitazone Medication (DREAM) study rosiglitazone was highly effective at reducing the progression to diabetes, but a non-significant increase in cardiovascular events was observed (see also Chapter 2).

1.4 **Insulin resistance and the metabolic syndrome**

Insulin resistance (or reduced insulin sensitivity) is established as a key part of type 2 diabetes when combined with beta-cell dysfunction, and more than 90% of patients are insulin resistant. A major advance in the understanding of insulin resistance came with the seminal work of Reaven, who made two key observations:

1. Resistance to insulin-stimulated glucose uptake is present in the majority of patients with impaired glucose tolerance and type 2 diabetes. He suggested that deterioration of glucose tolerance could only be prevented if the beta-cell is able to increase insulin secretion and maintain chronic hyperinsulinaemia. When this cannot be achieved gross decompensation of glucose homeostasis occurs and diabetes develops.

2. He observed clustering of risk factors for coronary heart disease in individual subjects, including hyperinsulinaemia, impaired glucose tolerance or diabetes, increased plasma triglyceride concentration, decreased HDL cholesterol concentration, and hypertension. He suggested that these might be causally linked by insulin resistance and hyperinsulinaemia, and referred to the cluster as 'Syndrome X'.

Others have referred to this as 'Reaven's syndrome', 'insulin resistance syndrome', or 'metabolic syndrome'. Whether there is a causal link or not, it is clear that insulin resistance is associated with other cardiovascular risk factors such as hyperglycaemia, hypertension, and dyslipidaemia. It is unclear why some individuals are insulin resistant, but genetic and environmental factors have both been implicated. In particular, physical inactivity and obesity are associated with insulin resistance, but not all obese persons are insulin resistant.

There are several methods of measuring insulin resistance for research purposes, but none are available in routine clinical practice. Several definitions of the metabolic syndrome are available based on clinical measures (Table 1.5).

Table 1.5 Definitions of the metabolic syndrome		
IDF 2005	**NCEP/ATPIII 2001**	**WHO 1999**
Abdominal obesity plus two or more risk factors	At least three risk factors	Diabetes/IGT/ insulin resistance plus two or more risk factors
Waist circumference ≥90cm (m), ≥80cm (f)	Waist circumference ≥102cm (m), ≥88cm (f)	BMI ≥30kg/m², and/or waist hip ratio >0.9 (m), >0.85 (f)
Blood pressure ≥130/≥85mmHg	Blood pressure ≥130/≥85mmHg	Blood pressure ≥140/≥90mmHg, or on medication
Fasting glucose ≥5.6mmol/L or pre-existing diabetes	Fasting glucose ≥6.1mmol/L or on medication for diabetes	Diabetes, impaired glucose tolerance or insulin resistance
Triglycerides ≥1.7mmol/L	Triglycerides ≥1.7mmol/L	Triglycerides ≥1.7mmol/L and/or HDL cholesterol <0.91mmol/L (m), <1.01mmol/L (f)
HDL cholesterol <1.04mmol/L (m), <1.3mmol/L (f)	HDL cholesterol <1.04mmol/L (m), <1.3mmol/L (f)	Urinary albumin excretion rate ≥20µg/min
Notes: m = male, f = female.		

The metabolic syndrome is a strong predictor of subsequent diabetes in non-diabetic individuals. A few recent studies have shown that insulin resistance in patients with type 2 diabetes is associated with increased cardiovascular risk, independent of other risk factors, but this is controversial.

The metabolic syndrome is not at present a separate target for treatment in patients with diabetes or in non-diabetic subjects, but the presence of the metabolic syndrome may influence the choice of drugs used for the treatment of hyperglycaemia or hypertension.

1.5 **Type 1 diabetes**

Prior to the discovery and clinical use of insulin in the 1920s, patients with type 1 diabetes survived around 1 year from the time of diagnosis. Death was caused by infection or severe metabolic acidosis. Initial hopes were that the widespread use of insulin would be a cure for this debilitating and fatal disease. It was soon clear that patients with type 1 diabetes on insulin therapy were surviving, but that their long-term outlook was poor because of the accelerated development of CHD. The relative risk of the development of CHD is greatly increased, but as type 1 diabetes affects a younger age group the absolute risk remains low (Figure 1.4).

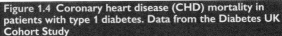

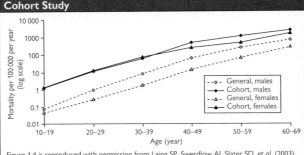

Figure 1.4 Coronary heart disease (CHD) mortality in patients with type 1 diabetes. Data from the Diabetes UK Cohort Study

Figure 1.4 is reproduced with permission from Laing SP, Swerdlow AJ, Slater SD, *et al.* (2003). *Diabetologia*, **46**: 760–5.

Because the event rate is lower, and many epidemiological studies combine type 1 and type 2 diabetes, it has been harder to identify what might be cardiovascular risk factors in patients with type 1 diabetes. Observations from the Pittsburgh Epidemiology of Diabetes Complications study have shown associations between incident CHD events and blood pressure, lipids, white cell count, renal disease, and peripheral vascular disease, with inverse associations with estimated glucose disposal rate and physical activity. Many of these are components of the metabolic syndrome, suggesting that the metabolic syndrome may have an important role in the pathophysiology of cardiovascular disease in type 1 diabetes.

1.6 Pathology of heart disease in diabetes

The pathology of CHD in diabetes is described in Chapter 5. When CHD develops it is more severe, with more left main stem disease and more triple vessel disease than in non-diabetic subjects, and coronary artery calcification is more extensive. The disease is also more diffuse, affecting proximal and distal segments of an affected artery, which has implications for coronary interventions (see Chapter 7). The development of collateral vessels is also reduced.

In addition to CHD, there is a 'diabetic cardiomyopathy' that can impair systolic emptying or diastolic filling of the left ventricle, and along with CHD contributes to the high prevalence of chronic heart failure in people with diabetes (Chapter 8).

1.7 **Conclusions**

Cardiovascular disease is a common cause of morbidity and mortality in people with diabetes, and several risk factors for the development of cardiovascular disease in diabetes are identified. There are no randomized control trials or systematic reviews of smoking cessation specifically in people with diabetes, and it is assumed that people with diabetes are likely to benefit from smoking cessation at least as much as people without diabetes. There are now multiple therapies that can be used to reduce cardiovascular risk in people with diabetes (Box 1.1). If we are going to obtain the greatest benefit and wish to reduce polypharmacy, we should concentrate on the use of interventions that have a proven evidence base.

> **Box 1.1 Interventions to reduce cardiovascular risk in people with type 2 diabetes**
>
> Treatment of hyperglycaemia
> * Metformin
> * Pioglitazone
>
> Treatment of dyslipidaemia
> * Statins
>
> Treatment of hypertension
> * Multiple antihypertensive drugs
>
> Antiplatelet drugs
> * Aspirin and/or clopidogrel for established cardiovascular disease

11

Key references

Chiasson JL, Josse RG, Gomis R, Hanefeld M, Karasik A, Laakso M. For the STOP-NIDDM Trial Research Group (2003). Acarbose treatment and the risk of cardiovascular disease and hypertension in patients with impaired glucose tolerance: the STOP-NIDDM trial. *Journal of the American Medical Association,* **290**: 486–94.

Evans JM, Wang J, Morris AD (2002). Comparison of cardiovascular risk between patients with type 2 diabetes and those who had had a myocardial infarction: cross sectional and cohort studies. *British Medical Journal,* **324**: 939–42.

Haffner SM, Lehto S, Ronnemaa T, Pyorala K, Laakso M (1998). Mortality from coronary heart disease in subjects with type 2 diabetes and in nondiabetic subjects with and without prior myocardial infarction. *New England Journal of Medicine,* **339**: 229–34.

Juutilainen A, Lehto S, Ronnemaa T, Pyorala K, Laakso M (2005). Type 2 diabetes as a 'coronary heart disease equivalent': an 18-year prospective population-based study in Finnish subjects. *Diabetes Care*, **28**: 2901–7.

Knowler WC, Barrett-Connor E, *et al.*, the Diabetes Prevention Program Research Group. (2002). Reduction in the incidence of type 2 diabetes with lifestyle intervention or metformin. *New England Journal of Medicine*, **346**: 393–403.

Laing SP, Swerdlow AJ, Slater SD, *et al.*, (2003). Mortality from heart disease in a cohort of 23,000 patients with insulin-treated diabetes. *Diabetologia*, **46**: 760–5.

Reaven GM (1988). Banting lecture 1988. Role of insulin resistance in human disease. *Diabetes*, **37**: 1595–607.

Tuomilehto J, Lindstrom J, Eriksson JG, *et al.*, for the Finnish Diabetes Prevention Study Group (2001). Prevention of type 2 diabetes mellitus by changes in lifestyle among subjects with impaired glucose tolerance. *New England Journal of Medicine*, **344**: 1343–50.

Chapter 2

Hyperglycaemia and weight management

Miles Fisher

Key points

- Intensive insulin therapy in patients with type 1 diabetes reduces cardiovascular outcomes on long-term follow-up.
- In patients with type 2 diabetes, tight glycaemic control does not significantly reduce macrovascular outcomes, but metformin reduces myocardial infarctions (MIs), separate from an effect on glycaemia.
- Pioglitazone reduces recurrent MIs and strokes in type 2 diabetic patients with established cardiovascular disease, but may cause fluid retention.
- Newer anti-diabetic drugs have some favourable effects on cardiovascular risk factors.
- In patients with type 2 diabetes anti-obesity drugs reduce weight and have some favourable effects on cardiovascular risk factors.

2.1 Management of glycaemia in type 1 diabetes

2.1.1 Diabetes Control and Complications Trial

The Diabetes Control and Complications Trial (DCCT) was established to prove that the intensive control of glycaemia, mimicking the pattern of physiological insulin secretion, reduced diabetic complications in patients with type 1 diabetes. Patients were randomized to intensive insulin therapy administered with an external insulin pump or by three or more daily insulin injections and guided by frequent blood-glucose monitoring, or to conventional therapy with one or two daily insulin injections. The patients were followed up for a mean of 6.5 years.

Intensive insulin therapy significantly reduced the risk of the development or progression of retinopathy, and reductions were also seen in the occurrence of microalbuminuria, macroalbuminuria, clinical neuropathy, and autonomic neuropathy. The chief adverse events associated with intensive insulin therapy were weight gain and an increase in severe hypoglycaemia.

The effects of intensive insulin therapy in the DCCT on cardiovascular risk factors are described in Box 2.1. The number of combined major cardiovascular events was almost twice as high in the conventionally treated group (40 events) as in the intensive-treatment group (23 events), but the difference was not statistically significant.

Box 2.1 Effects of intensive insulin therapy on cardiovascular risk factors in DCCT

- Reduced fasting, pre- and post-prandial hyperglycaemia
- Reduced HbA1c
- Reduced total and calculated LDL cholesterol
- Reduced triglycerides
- Increased development of low HDL cholesterol (secondary intervention cohort)
- Increased systolic blood pressure
- No difference in diastolic blood pressure
- No difference in smoking habits
- Increased body weight
- Increased development of raised waist-to-hip ratios
- Reduced microalbuminuria
- Reduced macroalbuminuria.

2.1.2 **Epidemiology of Diabetes Interventions and Complications study**

At the end of the DCCT, patients were returned to the care of their usual doctor, and patients in the conventional treatment group were offered intensified insulin regimens. Ninety-three per cent of the DCCT subjects were subsequently followed up in the observational Epidemiology of Diabetes Interventions and Complications (EDIC) study. The HbA1c concentrations decreased in the group that was formerly conventionally treated, and HbA1c increased in the subjects who were previously intensively treated when they were no longer in the intensive study environment, and thereafter the HbA1c concentrations in the two groups were similar.

During the mean 17 years of total follow-up, 46 cardiovascular events occurred in 31 patients who had received intensive treatment in the DCCT, as compared with 98 events in 52 patients who had received conventional treatment. Intensive treatment reduced the risk of any cardiovascular event by 42% and the risk of non-fatal MI, stroke, or death from cardiovascular disease by 57% (Figure 2.1). The decrease in HbA1c values during the DCCT was significantly associated

Figure 2.1 Reductions in cardiovascular disease outcomes (a) and non-fatal myocardial infarction (MI), stroke, or cardiovascular death (b) in the DCCT/EDIC study

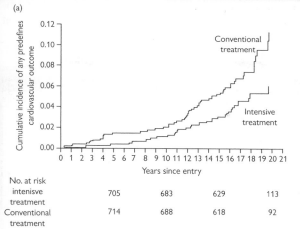

(a)

No. at risk				
intenisve treatment	705	683	629	113
Conventional treatment	714	688	618	92

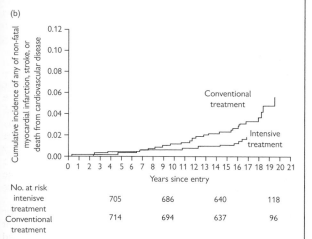

(b)

No. at risk				
intenisve treatment	705	686	640	118
Conventional treatment	714	694	637	96

with most of the beneficial effects of intensive treatment on the risk of cardiovascular disease, but microalbuminuria and albuminuria also had a role. The pathophysiological mechanisms responsible for the improvements in outcomes and for the prolonged effects of early intervention were unclear, and the authors referred to these as 'metabolic memory'.

- Other results of DCCT/EDIC are shown in Box 2.2.

Box 2.2 Effects of previous intensive insulin therapy on surrogate markers and endpoints in EDIC

- Reduced progression of retinopathy
- Reduced development and progression of nephropathy
- Reduced neuropathy
- Reduced incidence of hypertension
- Reduced progression of carotid intima-media thickness (CIMT)
- Reduced coronary artery calcification
- Reduced peripheral arterial calcification
- Lower resting heart rate.

2.1.3 **Cardiovascular effects of hypoglycaemia**

One of the chief adverse events associated with intensive insulin therapy in DCCT was an increase in severe hypoglycaemia, defined as requiring external assistance. Several subgroups defined by baseline characteristics had a particularly high risk of severe hypoglycaemia, including men, adolescents, subjects with no residual C-peptide secretion, and subjects with a previous history of hypoglycaemia. The physical consequences of hypoglycaemia that were reported in the DCCT included coma and seizures, and there were no reported cardiovascular consequences of hypoglycaemia.

Hypoglycaemia provokes an intense counter-regulatory hormonal response, including activation of the autonomic nervous system and the release of epinephrine (adrenaline) and norepinephrine (noradrenaline). The cardiovascular consequences of this include an increase in heart rate, an increase in systolic blood pressure, and a decrease in diastolic blood pressure, with widening of the pulse pressure and an increase in cardiac output. In a patient with coronary heart disease (CHD) these changes may be enough to cause angina and even myocardial infarction (MI) (Box 2.3).

Box 2.3 Cardiovascular consequences of hypoglycaemia

- **Physiological**
- Increased heart rate
- Increased systolic blood pressure, decreased diastolic blood pressure, widening of the pulse pressure
- Increased cardiac output
- Decreased peripheral vascular resistance
- Increased left ventricular ejection fraction.

- **Electrocardiography**
- Flattening or inversion of the T wave
- Lengthening of the QT interval
- ST segment depression.

- **Arrhythmias**
- Atrial and ventricular ectopics
- Sinus bradycardia
- Atrial fibrillation
- Ventricular tachycardia
- Ventricular fibrillation
- Asystole.

- **Pathological**
- Silent myocardial ischaemia
- Angina pectoris
- Myocardial infarction
- Cardiac arrest.

Intensive intravenous insulin treatment may be used to control hyperglycaemia following acute MI in diabetic and non-diabetic patients, and hypoglycaemia occurs in one-third of patients as a side effect. The changes in pulse and blood pressure are similar, and there are no reports of adverse consequences, arrhythmias, or myocardial ischaemia in that particular clinical situation.

2.2 Management of glycaemia in type 2 diabetes

2.2.1 Lifestyle measures in type 2 diabetes

Observational studies in diabetic and non-diabetic subjects indicate an association between reduced physical activity and subsequent cardiovascular outcomes. The pathophysiology of type 2 diabetes includes beta-cell dysfunction and insulin resistance. Lifestyle measures, including diet, increased physical activity, and behaviour modification, can reduce insulin resistance and improve glycaemic control and cardiovascular risk markers (reduced HbA1c, reduced systolic and diastolic blood pressure, reduced triglycerides, increased HDL cholesterol, reduced urinary albumin excretion), although to date studies have only followed patients for a few years.

2.2.2 Metformin and the United Kingdom Prospective Diabetes Study (UKPDS)

The United Kingdom Prospective Diabetes Study (UKPDS) tested the hypothesis that tight glycaemia control in type 2 diabetes would reduce microvascular and macrovascular complications, and that there might be advantages of certain agents. This was because an earlier study from the United States had suggested an increase in mortality with the sulphonylurea tolbutamide. The principal comparisons were between a group of patients who received conventional treatment and a group of patients who received intensive treatment based on therapy with a sulphonylurea or insulin. A small subgroup of overweight patients was randomized to metformin.

In the intensively treated group tight control reduced microvascular endpoints, in particular the need for photocoagulation for diabetic retinopathy. There was a statistically insignificant reduction in MIs.

The main side effects of sulphonylureas in UKPDS were weight gain and hypoglycaemia, and there was no evidence of adverse cardiovascular effects. Sulphonylureas and the newer non-sulphonylurea insulin secretagogues, repaglinide and nateglinide, increase basal and postprandial insulin secretion by closing the K_{ATP} channel in pancreatic beta-cells. In the heart some of these drugs antagonize K_{ATP} channels, which are important in ischaemic pre- and post-conditioning, and in theory could increase the amount of myocardial damage at the time of MI. This has been demonstrated in animal models of infarction and laboratory experiments, but clinical studies have not established a link between sulphonylurea treatment before the acute MI and poor outcomes.

In overweight patients in UKPDS, metformin significantly reduced MIs, cardiovascular deaths, and all-cause mortality (Figure 2.2). The reductions could not be explained by any differences in HbA1c, as HbA1c was similar in overweight patients who received intensive treatment with insulin, sulphonylureas, or metformin, suggesting that these were due to some other effect of metformin. It was suggested that the beneficial effects of metformin on hepatic insulin resistance or on fibrinolysis might have been responsible for the reduction in MIs.

Figure 2.2 Clinical endpoints in the overweight patients in the UKPDS assigned intensive control with metformin, intensive control with sulphonylurea or insulin, or conventional control

Aggregate Endpoint	p for metformin vs other intensive	Patients with aggregate endpoints		Absolute risk (events per 1000 patient-years)		Log rank 2p	RR (95% CI) vs conventional
		Metformin or Intensive	Conventional	Metformin or Intensive	Conventional		
Any diabetes-related endpoint	p = 0.0084						
Metformin		98	160	29.8	43.3	0.0023	0.68 (0.53–0.87)
Intensive		350	160	40.1	43.3	0.46	0.93 (0.77–1.12)
Diabetes-related death	p = 0.11						
Metformin		28	55	7.5	12.7	0.017	0.58 (0.37–0.91)
Intensive		103	55	10.3	12.7	0.19	0.80 (0.58–1.11)
All-cause mortality	p = 0.021						
Metformin		50	89	13.6	20.6	0.011	0.64 (0.45–0.91)
Intensive		190	89	18.9	20.6	0.49	0.92 (0.71–1.18)
Myocardial infarction	p = 0.12						
Metformin		99	73	11.0	18.0	0.01	0.61 (0.41–0.89)
Intensive		139	73	14.4	18.0	0.11	0.79 (0.60–1.05)
Stroke	p = 0.032						
Metformin		12	23	3.3	5.5	0.13	0.59 (0.29–1.18)
Intensive		60	23	6.2	5.5	0.60	1.14 (0.70–1.84)
Peripheral vascular disease	p = 0.62						
Metformin		6	9	1.6	2.1	0.57	0.74 (0.28–2.09)
Intensive		12	9	1.2	2.1	0.18	0.56 (0.24–1.33)
Microvascular	p = 0.39						
Metformin		24	38	6.7	9.2	0.19	0.71 (0.43–1.19)
Intensive		74	38	7.7	9.2	0.38	0.84 (0.57–1.24)

Figure 2.2 is reproduced with permission from UK Prospective Diabetes Study (UKPDS) Group. (1998), *Lancet*, **352**: 854–65.

CHAPTER 2 **Hyperglycaemia and weight management**

There have been several other publications from the UKPDS that have given useful information about cardiovascular risk in type 2 diabetes (Box 2.4).

> ### Box 2.4 Cardiovascular results from the UKPDS
>
> - **Principal results**
> - Metformin significantly reduced MIs, diabetes-related deaths, and all-cause mortality.
>
> - **Other important cardiovascular results**
> - Intensive blood-glucose control with metformin was cost-effective in overweight patients with type 2 diabetes.
> - The effects of glycaemia and blood pressure reduction on the risk of complications was additive.
> - The presence of the metabolic syndrome at baseline identified patients at greater risk of macrovascular but not microvascular complications.
> - Insulin sensitivity at diagnosis was not associated with subsequent cardiovascular disease.
> - After adjusting for conventional cardiovascular risk factors the risk of MI was similar in white and South Asian patients and lower in Afro-Caribbean subjects.

2.2.3 Thiazolidinediones or 'glitazones'

The thiazolidinediones rosiglitazone and pioglitazone are agonists for peroxisome-proliferator-activated receptor gamma (PPAR gamma) in adipose tissue, liver, and skeletal muscle, reducing insulin resistance and leading to a reduction of blood-glucose concentration. When used in man they have potentially beneficial effects on several cardio-vascular risk factors (Box 2.5), including reductions in blood pressure and C-reactive protein (CRP). Both glitazones cause weight gain. In double blind comparator studies it has been shown that the effects on lipids are different. In particular, pioglitazone reduces triglycerides and increases HDL cholesterol, whereas rosiglitazone increases total and LDL cholesterol concentrations.

> **Box 2.5 Effects of glitazones on cardiovascular risk factors**
>
> • **Potentially beneficial**
> • Improved glycaemia control
> • Reduced blood pressure
> • Reduced microalbuminuria
> • Reduced C-reactive protein
> • Reduced small, dense LDL (especially pioglitazone)
> • Increased HDL cholesterol (especially pioglitazone)
> • Reduced triglycerides (pioglitazone).
>
> • **Potentially adverse**
> • Weight gain
> • Increased total and LDL cholesterol (rosiglitazone).

Glitazones cause the retention of fluid through mechanisms in the distal tubules of the kidney. This may manifest itself as weight gain or ankle oedema. In a patient with early left ventricular systolic function, or diastolic dysfunction, this fluid retention can unmask heart failure. Glitazones are contraindicated in patients with a history of heart failure (see also Chapter 8).

The PROspective pioglitAzone Clinical Trial In macroVascular Events (PROactive) study examined the effects of pioglitazone on cardiovascular events in patients with type 2 diabetes and existing cardiovascular disease. There was a statistically insignificant reduction of 10% in the primary endpoint, which comprised disease endpoints (death, MI, stroke, acute coronary syndromes) and procedural end-points (coronary revascularization, leg amputation, leg revascularization). A main secondary endpoint of cardiovascular death, MI or stroke, was significantly reduced by 16%. Subgroup analysis of patients who had a previous MI or strokes showed further reductions in MIs and strokes, respectively.

A recent meta-analysis of cardiovascular events in patients treated with pioglitazone confirmed a significant reduction in all-cause mortality, MIs, and strokes with pioglitazone in people with type 2 diabetes (Figure 2.3).

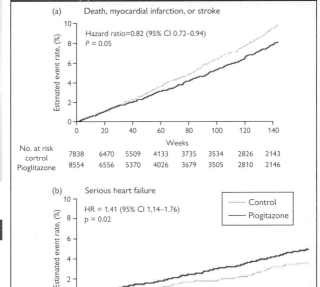

Figure 2.3 **Cardiovascular end points in the pioglitazone meta-analysis, including death, MI, or stroke (a) and serious heart failure (b)**

(a) Death, myocardial infarction, or stroke

Hazard ratio=0.82 (95% CI 0.72–0.94)
P = 0.05

Estimated event rate, (%)

Weeks

No. at risk								
control	7838	6470	5509	4133	3735	3534	2826	2143
Pioglitazone	8554	6556	5370	4026	3679	3505	2810	2146

(b) Serious heart failure

HR = 1.41 (95% CI 1,14–1.76)
p = 0.02

—— Control
—— Pioglitazone

Estimated event rate, (%)

Weeks

7836	6485	5544	4181	3803	3622	2911	2230
8554	6563	5388	4052	3696	3527	2827	2163

Figure 2.3 is reproduced with permission from Lincoff AM, Wolski K, Nicholls SJ, Nissen SE (2007). *Journal of American Medical Association*, **298**: 1180–8.

The effects of rosiglitazone on cardiovascular outcomes are controversial. A meta-analysis was performed of trials where rosiglitazone was given for at least 24 weeks, there was a comparable group not receiving rosiglitazone, and there was outcome data for MI and death from cardiovascular causes. In the rosiglitazone group there were 86 MIs in 15 560 subjects, and in the comparator group there were 72 MIs in 12 283 subjects, giving an odds ratio of 1.43 for MI (95% CI 1.03–1.99; P=0.03) with an insignificant rise in cardiovascular deaths. These results were similar to previous meta-analyses performed by the manufacturer of rosiglitazone, and by the U.S. Federal Drug Administration (FDA).

The Rosiglitazone Evaluated for Cardiac Outcomes and Regulation of glycaemia in Diabetes (RECORD) study was prospectively established to examine the cardiovascular effects of rosiglitazone. An interim analysis was published following the meta-analysis, which highlights major deficiencies in study design. The study is open label and not double blind, and is a 'non-inferiority' study. Ten per cent of patients have already been lost to follow-up, and the primary event rate is much lower than predicted. There were no significant differences between the rosiglitazone group and the control group regarding MI and death from cardiovascular causes, but an increase in these could not be excluded. When these data are added to the meta-analysis there remains an increase in MIs with rosiglitazone.

2.2.4 **Acarbose**

Acarbose is an alpha-glucosidase inhibitor that inhibits digestion of polysaccharides from the small intestine, reducing post-prandial glucose concentrations. Meta-analysis of the effects of acarbose in patients with type 2 diabetes has given conflicting results. One meta-analysis suggested a reduction in cardiovascular events, whereas a Cochrane review suggested no evidence of any benefit for mortality and morbidity.

2.2.5 **Newer anti-diabetic drugs**

Therapies are now available that exploit the incretin effect for clinical benefit. Glucagon-like peptide-1 (GLP-1) is one of the main incretin hormones, but is rapidly degraded to inactive metabolites by the enzyme dipeptidyl pepitidase-4 (DPP-4). DPP-4 inhibitors are oral drugs that inhibit the action of DPP-4 and increase the amount of endogenous GLP-1 and glucose-dependent insulinotropic peptide (GIP). In clinical use sitagliptin, the first available DPP-4 inhibitor, reduces HbA1c, has no effect on body weight, and no discernable effect on cardiovascular risk markers.

The alternative approach is to use synthetic analogues of GLP-1 that are resistant to degradation by DPP-4. Exenatide is an incretin mimetic that was first identified in the saliva of the Gila monster. It is given twice daily by subcutaneous injection, and increases glucose-dependent promotion of insulin secretion, inhibits glucagon secretion, delays gastric emptying, and suppresses appetite, with associated weight loss of 4–5kg over 1 year. This weight loss has in turn been associated with reductions in diastolic blood pressure, triglycerides, and increases in HDL cholesterol.

The occurrence of GLP-1 receptors in cardiac tissue and the central nervous system has stimulated investigation of GLP-1 and cardiac effects in animals, but as yet the relevance to humans is not certain.

2.2.6 **Blood glucose targets**

In the UKPDS the mean HbA1c concentration in the intensive treatment group was 7.0%. Two large multi-centre studies were set up to examine if a lower target HbA1c would reduce cardiovascular events and have recently reported. The Action to Control Cardiovascular Risk in Diabetes (ACCORD) Study aimed to reduce HbA1c to non-diabetic levels of less than 6.0%. The study was stopped early because of an increase in total mortality in the intensive treatment group, and the HbA1c that was reached was 6.5%. There were significant increases in severe hypoglycaemia and weight gain in the intensive treatment group compared to the standard therapy group. Rosiglitazone was the glitazone of choice in the study, and investigators could not establish a link with any particular treatment or with hypoglycaemia, but undetected hypoglycaemia provoking arrhythmias is the most likely explanation for the findings.

The Action in Diabetes and Vascular disease: preterAx and diamicroN-MR Controlled Evaluation (ADVANCE) study aimed to obtain a target HbA1c of 6.5% in the intensive group, and this was finally achieved at the end of the study, whereas in ACCORD the lower HbA1c was achieved within the first four months. There was a significant reduction in microvascular events with more intensive therapy in ADVANCE, but there was no effect, either beneficial or harmful, on macrovascular events or mortality. Hypoglycaemia was not a common problem in ADVANCE. On present evidence a target HbA1c of <7.0% and not lower than 6.5% seems prudent."

2.3 **Anti-obesity drugs**

2.3.1 **Principles of drug therapy for obesity**

Anti-obesity agents can have indirect effects on insulin resistance and hyperglycaemia, mediated by weight loss. Treatments include drugs that decrease nutrient absorption, and drugs that decrease food intake by reducing appetite or increasing satiety. Appetite suppressants work by changing the availability of neurotransmitters. In the past noradrenergic agents were used, but they are no longer recommended because of the risk of abuse. Fenfluramine, a drug that stimulated the release of serotonin and inhibited its reuptake, was withdrawn because of associations with valvular heart disease and pulmonary hypertension.

2.3.2 **Orlistat**

Orlistat is a gastric and pancreatic lipase inhibitor that reduces dietary fat absorption, and when used in addition to other anti-diabetic drugs, including metformin, sulphonylureas, and insulin, it has resulted in increased weight loss and a reduction in HbA1c, blood pressure, total and LDL cholesterol, with a slight reduction in HDL cholesterol (Table 2.1).

Table 2.1 Effects of anti-obesity drugs on cardiovascular risk factors in patients with type 2 diabetes			
	Orlistat	Sibutramine	Rimonabant
Weight	Decreased	Decreased	Decreased
Waist circumference	Decreased	Decreased	Decreased
HbA1c	Decreased	Decreased	Decreased
Systolic blood pressure	Decreased	Increased	Decreased
Diastolic blood pressure	Decreased	Increased	Insignificant decrease
Total cholesterol	Decreased	No change	No change
LDL cholesterol	Decreased	No change	No change
HDL cholesterol	Decreased	Increased	Increased
Triglycerides	No change	Decreased	Decreased

2.3.3 Sibutramine

Sibutramine inhibits the reuptake of norepinephrine (noradrenaline) and serotonin, promoting satiety and weight loss. It is associated with small increases in pulse and blood pressure, and should be discontinued if blood pressure exceeds 145/90mmHg or if diastolic pressure rises by more than 10mmHg. Controlled hypertension is not a contraindication to its use. Meta-analysis of the effects of sibutramine in type 2 diabetes showed reductions in HbA1c and triglycerides, with increases in HDL cholesterol, and no change in total and LDL cholesterol (Table 2.1). The effects on MI, stroke, and cardiovascular mortality are being explored in the ongoing Sibutramine Cardiovascular Outcomes (SCOUT) study, which includes subjects with type 2 diabetes.

2.3.4 Rimonabant

Rimonabant is an appetite suppressant that promotes weight loss through blockade of the type 1 cannabinoid receptor. In diabetic patients, the use of this agent has been associated with increased weight loss, reductions in HbA1c, improvements in lipids, and reductions in blood pressure (Table 2.1). Part of the metabolic effect may be secondary to loss of weight, and part due to blockade of cannabinoid receptors in adipose tissue. The main side effect is an increase in depression. Cardiovascular outcome studies and studies in subjects with pre-diabetes are currently underway.

Key references

Action to Control Cardiovascular Risk in Diabetes Study Group (2008). Effects of intensive glucose lowering in type 2 diabetes. *New England Journal of Medicine*, **358**: 2545–59.

ADVANCE Collaborative Group (2008). Intensive blood glucose control and vascular outcomes in patients with type 2 diabetes. *New England Journal of Medicine*, **358**: 2560–72.

Diabetes Control and Complications Trial (DCCT) Research Group (1995). Effect of intensive diabetes management on macrovascular events and risk factors in the Diabetes Control and Complications Trial. *American. Journal of Cardiology*, **75**: 894–903.

Diabetes Control and Complications Trial/Epidemiology of Diabetes Interventions and Complications (DCCT/EDIC) Study Research Group (2005). Intensive diabetes treatment and cardiovascular disease in patients with type 1 diabetes. *New England Journal of Medicine*, **353**: 2643–53.

Dormandy JA, Charbonnel B, Eckland DJA, Erdmann E, Massi-Benedetti M, Moules IK, *et al.* on behalf of the PROactive investigators (2005). Secondary prevention of macrovascular events in patients with type 2 diabetes in the PROactive study (PROspective pioglitAzone Clinical Trial In macroVascular Events): a randomised controlled trial. *Lancet*, **366**: 1279–89.

Lincoff, AM, Wolski K, Nicholls SJ, Nissen SE (2007). Pioglitazone and risk of cardiovascular events in patients with type 2 diabetes mellitus: a meta-analysis of randomized trials. *Journal of American Medical Association*, **298**: 1180–8.

Nissen SE and Wolski K (2007). Effect of rosiglitazone on the risk of myocardial infarction and death from cardiovascular causes. *New England Journal of Medicine*, **356**: 2457–71.

Rucker D, Padwal R, Li SK, Curoni C, Lau DCW (2007). Long term pharmacotherapy for obesity and overweight: updated meta-analysis. *British Medical Journal*, **335**: 1194–9.

Scheen AJ, Finer N, Hollander P, Jensen MD, Van Gaal LF for the RIO-Diabetes Study Group (2006). Efficacy and tolerability of rimonabant in overweight or obese patients with type 2 diabetes: a randomised controlled study. *Lancet*, **368**: 1660–72.

UK Prospective Diabetes Study (UKPDS) Group (1998a). Intensive blood-glucose control with sulphonylureas or insulin compared with conventional treatment and risk of complications in patients with type 2 diabetes (UKPDS 33). *Lancet*, **352**: 837–53.

UK Prospective Diabetes Study (UKPDS) Group (1998b). Effect of intensive blood-glucose control with metformin on complications in overweight patients with type 2 diabetes (UKPDS 34). *Lancet*, **352**: 854–65.

Chapter 3

Diabetic dyslipidaemia

Miles Fisher

Key points

- The typical dyslipidaemia in type 2 diabetes and the metabolic syndrome comprises low-HDL cholesterol concentrations and raised triglycerides. Total and LDL cholesterol are not raised, but the proportion of atherogenic small dense LDL cholesterol is increased.

- In large studies statins have been proven to reduce cardiovascular events in people with diabetes who have known cardiovascular disease ('secondary prevention') and who have increased cardiovascular risk ('primary prevention').

- Larger doses of statins have further reduced cardio-vascular events in people with cardiovascular disease and diabetes compared to smaller doses, but with an increase in side effects and cost.

- Few studies have included patients with type 1 diabetes, and the clinical use of statins in patients with type 1 diabetes, and in younger patients with type 2 diabetes, is based on expert opinion extrapolated from older patients with type 2 diabetes.

- Fibrates reduce triglycerides and increase HDL cholesterol, but the results of large studies with fibrates in patients with diabetes have been disappointing and mostly negative.

3.1 Description of the dyslipidaemia of diabetes

Diabetes and dyslipidaemia are components of the metabolic syndrome. The typical dyslipdaemia of diabetes consists of low-HDL cholesterol concentrations, raised triglycerides, and an increase in the proportion of small, dense particles of LDL cholesterol, which are more atherogenic than larger LDL particles. There are associated abnormalities in other lipid sub-fractions and apolipoproteins (Box 3.1).

Box 3.1 Diabetic dyslipidaemia

Increased
- Triglycerides
- Apolipoprotein B
- Very low-density lipoproteins (VLDLs), especially VLDL1
- Triglyceride-rich remnants
- Small dense LDL
- Post-prandial lipaemia.

Decreased
- HDL cholesterol, especially HDL2
- Apolipoprotein A-1.

Epidemiological evidence has shown a strong association betwee levels of total and LDL cholesterol and vascular events, an invers relationship between HDL concentrations and vascular events, and some epidemiological studies raised triglycerides were a risk facto for vascular events independent of low-HDL concentrations. Of th available lipid-regulating drugs, fibrates improve the lipid profil reducing triglycerides and increasing HDL cholesterol, but there limited evidence from clinical trials that this reduces cardiovascul events, and most of the evidence is for statins.

3.2 Statins

Statins competitively inhibit 3-hydroy-3-methylglutaryl coenzyme (HMG CoA) reductase, reducing cholesterol synthesis in the live There is evidence of cardiovascular risk reduction with statins people with diabetes, both as primary and secondary prevention, ar for several different statins, suggesting a possible class effect (Box 3.2

Box 3.2 Evidence for benefits of statins in diabetic patients

Statins of proven benefit
- Stable coronary disease (simvastatin, pravastatin, atorvastatin)
- Patients without known vascular disease ('primary prevention') (simvastatin, atorvastatin)
- Acute coronary syndromes (atorvastatin)
- Following coronary artery bypass surgery (lovastatin)
- Following percutaneous coronary interventions (fluvastatin)
- Following stroke (simvastatin, atorvastatin).

Statin studies negative
- Chronic renal failure
- Haemodialysis patients
- Chronic heart failure.

ot every study has been positive, and there are studies where the nefit in people with diabetes has not reached statistical significance, ossibly because of small numbers in the subgroup. In one study in der patients the number of events was insignificantly increased in abetic subjects treated with pravastatin compared to diabetic patients eated with placebo, although the study overall showed significant rdiovascular benefit from pravastatin.

2.1 **Older statins—simvastatin and pravastatin**

itial statin trials were in patients with established coronary heart sease (CHD) and raised total cholesterols, using simvastatin and -avastatin. Subgroup analysis of diabetic subgroups demonstrated milar relative risk reductions for total mortality, cardiovascular mor- lity, and major coronary events, and as the event rate was higher in eople with diabetes the absolute risk reduction was greater.

The Scandinavian Simvastatin Survival Study (4S) examined the fects of simvastatin in patients with angina or previous myocardial farction (MI) and raised total cholesterol. Most patients received)mg of simvastatin, but around one-third had the dose increased to)mg. Simvastatin reduced the primary endpoint of total mortality, id there was a significant reduction in 'major coronary events' CHD-related death and non-fatal MI). There were two post hoc ibgroup analyses of diabetic patients. The first examined patients 'ith known diabetes at the start of the study, and revealed significant eductions in major coronary events. The second added people agnosed using the new WHO criteria, and the reduction in major oronary events was similar. There have been several other publica- ons from 4S that have given useful information about cardiovascular sk in type 2 diabetes (Box 3.3).

Results similar to 4S were found using pravastatin for secondary revention in the Cholesterol and Recurrent Events (CARE) trial and e Long-Term Intervention with Pravastatin in Ischaemic Disease (LIPID) ial. The West of Scotland Coronary Prevention Study (WOSCOPS) 'ith pravastatin was the first study to demonstrate reduced cardiovas- ular events in subjects without MI, but WOSCOPS contained only 76 nown diabetic patients (1%); therefore subgroup analysis of diabetic atients was not possible.

Box 3.3 Results of the 4S study

Principal results

- In patients with diabetes and CHD simvastatin significantly reduced major CHD events and insignificantly reduced total mortality.

Other results from 4S

- For patients with diabetes estimates of cost per life-year gained were well within the range generally considered to be cost-effective.
- In patients with impaired fasting glucose, simvastatin reduced major coronary events, revascularizations, total and coronary mortality.
- Simvastatin significantly reduced cardiovascular disease-related hospitalizations and total hospital days for patients with normal fasting glucose, impaired fasting glucose, and diabetes, and significantly reduced length of stay for people with diabetes.
- Non-diabetic patients with or without the metabolic syndrome benefited from simvastatin. The absolute benefit was greater in patients with the metabolic syndrome because they had a higher absolute risk.

Some further interesting data about diabetes emerged from follow up of the WOSCOPS cohort:

- Non-diabetic subjects who received pravastatin had a 30% reduction in the chance of developing new onset diabetes.
- Baseline predictors of the development of new onset diabetes included body mass index, fasting triglyceride, fasting glucose, and C-reactive protein (CRP) concentrations.
- Prior to conversion to diabetes converters had an increase in ALT and triglycerides, suggesting hepatic fat accumulation as a contributing factor.

Later statin trials were performed in subjects with 'normal' cholesterol concentrations, patients with other forms of vascular disease, and diabetic patients without known vascular disease. The Heart Protection Study (HPS) addressed the possible benefit of simvastatin 40mg in 20 536 subjects who would not have been included in the early coronary studies. There were 5963 diabetic subjects (29% of the total), mostly with type 2 diabetes. This was the first study to demonstrate a reduction in strokes with statins in addition to the reduction in coronary events in people with diabetes (Figure 3.1). A total of 2912 diabetic patients (49% of diabetic subjects) had no prior occlusive vascular disease (primary prevention), and simvastatin significantly reduced the primary endpoint of first major cardiovascular event from 13% down to 9% in this subgroup.

Of the older statins, there is a large evidence base for the use of simvastatin and pravastatin for both primary and secondary prevention in people with diabetes.

Lovastatin and fluvastatin have been shown to be of benefit in diabetic patients, following coronary artery bypass grafting and percutaneous coronary interventions (Box 3.2). Together these results suggest that the benefits of statins are a probably a class effect.

3.2.2 Newer statins—atorvastatin

The Collaborative AtoRvastatin Diabetes Study (CARDS) was the first study which assessed the benefits of cholesterol reduction solely in a cohort of subjects with diabetes, and randomized 2838 participants with type 2 diabetes and no previous cardiovascular disease to atorvastatin 10mg or placebo.

CARDS was stopped early because of a significant reduction of 37% in the composite primary endpoint of 'major cardiovascular events', which comprised all acute CHD events, including resuscitated cardiac arrest, coronary revascularization procedures, and stroke. The largest benefit was seen in stroke prevention with a 48% risk reduction. These results were seen with initial LDL levels both above and below the median. Further analysis of the data showed that atorvastatin was cost-effective, significantly reduced major cardiovascular events as early as 18 months after initiation of treatment, with a significant reduction in CHD events as early as one year, and was effective in patients aged 65–75.

Figure 3.1 Reductions in vascular events with simvastatin 40mg in people with and without diabetes in the Heart Protection Study (HPS)

Major vascular event and prior disease group	Simvastatin-allocated (10 269)	Placebo-allocated (10 267)	Event rate ratio (95% CI)	P-value for heterogeneity
Major coronary events				
Diabetes	279 (9.4%)	377 (12.6%)		
No diabetes	619 (8.5%)	835 (11.5%)		
Subtotal: coronary event	898 (8.7%)	1212 (11.8%)	0.73 (0.67–0.79) P<0.0001	1.0
Strokes				
Diabetes	149 (5.0%)	193 (6.5%)		
No diabetes	295 (4.0%)	392 (5.4%)		
Subtotal: stroke	444 (4.3%)	585 (5.7%)	0.75 (0.66–0.85) P<0.0001	0.9
Revascularisations				
Diabetes	260 (8.7%)	309 (10.4%)		
No diabetes	679 (9.3%)	896 (12.3%)		
Subtotal: revascularisation	939 (9.1%)	1205 (11.7%)	0.76 (0.70–0.83) P<0.0001	0.3
Major vascular events				
Diabetes	601 (20.2%)	748 (25.1%)		
No diabetes	1432 (19.6%)	1837 (25.2%)		
Any major vascular event	2033 (19.8%)	2585 (25.2%)	0.76 (0.72–0.81) P<0.0001	0.6

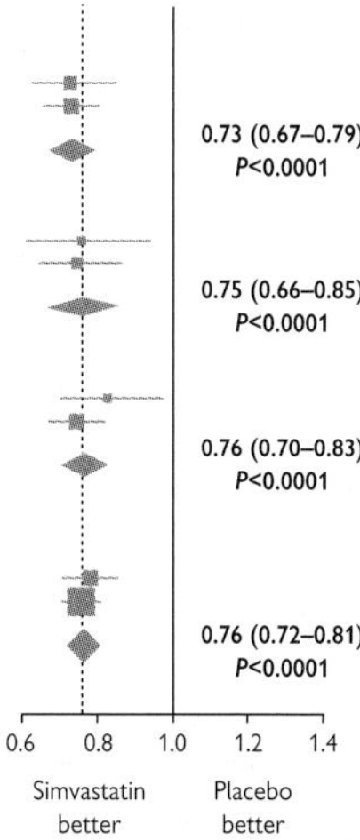

0.6 0.8 1.0 1.2 1.4
Simvastatin better   Placebo better

Figure 3.1 is reproduced with permission from Heart Protection Study Collaborative Group (2003). *Lancet*, 361: 2005–16.

3.2.3 **Rosuvastatin**

Rosuvastatin is one of the newest and most potent statins, and has been shown in short-term trials to be more effective than atorvastatin at reducing total and LDL cholesterol, and CRP in people with diabetes. Rosuvastatin should be considered where diabetic patients have failed to reach targets with one of the other statins (Table 3.1).

3.2.4 **Ezetimibe**

An alternative approach if the patient fails to reach target is the addition of ezetimibe. Ezetimibe is the first cholesterol absorption inhibitor and therefore has a mode of action that is complementary to statins. It has been shown to lead to substantial reductions in cholesterol when added to statins in patients with diabetes. At present there is no double-blind, randomized endpoint trial to support its use.

3.2.5 **Higher doses of statins**

Observations have suggested that lower total or LDL cholesterol concentrations are associated with lower vascular events rates, leading to the hypothesis that higher doses of statins, causing greater reductions in cholesterol, would lead to greater reductions in vascular events. Most of the comparisons have used high-dose atorvastatin, and further reductions in cardiovascular events have been demonstrated, including in diabetic subgroups. This includes patients with acute coronary syndromes, stable CHD, and strokes.

Table 3.1 Lipid-lowering therapy in diabetes		
	Primary prevention	**Secondary prevention**
Which patients?	All patients >40 years of age, high risk <40 years	All diabetic patients
Which statin?	Simvastatin 40mg, or atorvastatin 10mg	Simvastatin 40mg, atorvastatin 80mg if acute coronary syndrome
What total cholesterol target?	<5.0mmol/L	<4.0mmol/L
What LDL cholesterol target?	<3.0mmol/L	<2.0mmol/L
What to do if not to target?	Switch to more potent statin, e.g., atorvastatin 40mg, or add ezetimibe 10mg	Switch to more potent statin, e.g., atorvastatin 80mg, or add ezetimibe 10mg

The Pravastatin or Atorvastatin Evaluation and Infection Therapy-Thrombolysis in Myocardial Infraction 22 (PROVE-IT TIMI 22) trial compared 40mg of pravastatin versus 80mg of atorvastatin in patients with recent acute coronary syndromes. At the start of the study they had modestly elevated total and LDL cholesterol levels of 4.7 and 2.7mmol/L, respectively. After a mean follow-up period of 24 months the atorvastatin group achieved a 32% reduction in LDL cholesterol (2.7 to 1.6mmol/L) compared to minor reductions seen with pravastatin (2.7 to 2.4mmol/L). There was a 16% reduction in the primary endpoint of time to first major cardiovascular event, including death from any cause, MI, unstable angina, stroke, and revascularization procedures. There were 978 subjects with diabetes in the study (23%). There was a non-significant reduction in the time to first major cardiovascular event within this subgroup, probably reflecting the relatively small number of patients with diabetes. Acute coronary events were significantly reduced by 25% (Figure 3.2).

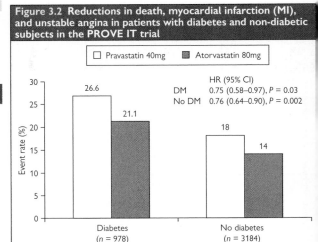

Figure 3.2 Reductions in death, myocardial infarction (MI), and unstable angina in patients with diabetes and non-diabetic subjects in the PROVE IT trial

Figure 3.2 is reproduced with permission from Ahmed S, Cannon CP, Murphy SA, Braunwald E (2006). *European Heart Journal,* **27**: 2323–9.

The Treatment to New Targets (TNT) study looked at atorvastatin 10mg versus 80mg in patients with stable CHD. This was a large, open label study, which randomized 10001 patients with CHD, 15% of whom had diabetes. By the end of the run-in period the mean LDL in both patient groups was 2.6mmol/L. This was reduced further to a mean of 2.0mmol/L in the 80mg atorvastatin group and resulted in a significant 22% relative risk reduction in the primary endpoint of major cardiovascular events, which included death from CHD or stroke, non-fatal or procedural MI, resuscitated cardiac arrest, or non-fatal stroke.

In diabetic subjects there was a 25% relative risk reduction in major cardiovascular events, which was seen for all quintiles of age, initial LDL or duration of diabetes, and in patients with HbA1c < or > 7% (Figure 3.3). There were too few subjects to see significant reductions in most of the secondary endpoints, although there was a significant reduction in the time to cerebrovascular events and time to cardiovascular events with high-dose atorvastatin.

In both PROVE IT and TNT the main side effect of higher-dose statins was an increase in abnormalities of liver function tests.

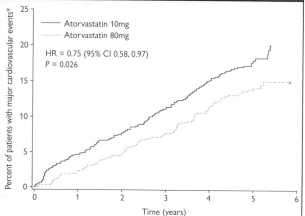

Figure 3.3 Further reductions in cardiovascular events in people with diabetes in the Treating to New Targets (TNT) study

Figure 3.3 is reproduced with permission from Shepherd J, Barter P, Carmena R, Deedwania P, Fruchart JC, Haffner S, et al. for the Treating to New Targets Investigators (2006). *Diabetes Care*, **29**: 1220–6.

3.2.6 **Systematic reviews and meta-analyses**

There are several systematic reviews and meta-analyses of statin studies in people with diabetes. In one meta-analysis comparing diabetic and non-diabetic subjects, it was demonstrated that lipids were reduced to a similar degree in both groups, but that diabetic patients benefited more in both primary and secondary prevention because of the greater absolute risk reduction.

The Cholesterol Treatment Trialists' (CTT) Collaborators performed a meta-analysis of cholesterol-lowering therapy in 18 686 people with diabetes in 14 randomized trials of statins. There was a 9% reduction in all-cause mortality per mmol/L reduction in LDL cholesterol, with a 21% reduction in major vascular events per mmol/L reduction in LDL cholesterol. There was some limited direct evidence of benefit in 1466 people with type 1 diabetes.

3.2.7 **Statins for lower-risk diabetic patients**

There were very few subjects with type 1 diabetes in the studies described earlier, and most subjects were middle-aged or elderly. Many guidelines suggest the use of statins in younger patients with diabetes, and suggest ways of identifying younger patients with diabetes who are at increased risk. These include using formal risk calculation, or use in patients with components of the metabolic syndrome (low-HDL cholesterol, raised triglycerides, hypertension) and a family history of CVD, retinopathy, or nephropathy.

3.2.8 **Cholesterol targets in diabetes**

Several different targets are set in different guidelines for cholesterol lowering in people with diabetes. Some include an 'audit' total cholesterol of 5mmol/L, and an LDL cholesterol of 3mmol/L. Scientific evidence supports the use of higher-dose statins to lower targets of 4mmol/L total cholesterol and 2mmol/L LDL cholesterol. This approach may not be cost-effective in diabetic patients without known cardiovascular disease, but is strongly recommended for patients with established cardiovascular disease, especially following acute coronary syndromes.

3.3 **Other lipid-lowering drugs**

3.3.1 **Fibrates**

Fibrates act through PPAR alpha, leading to increases in HDL cholesterol and reductions in triglycerides. In theory they should be more suitable to correct the dyslipidaemia of diabetes and reduce cardiovascular events, but the evidence for this is rather limited. Most of the clinical trials of fibrates in diabetes have been negative, and only gemfibrozil is of proven benefit in diabetic patients with CHD. Other studies have shown benefits with statins in similar groups of patients, and combination of gemfibrozil with a statin is contraindicated because of an increase in muscle side effects.

The recent Fenofibrate Intervention and Event Lowering in Diabetes (FIELD) study examined the effects of fenofibrate in people with diabetes, mostly without existing vascular disease. There was no effect of fenofibrate on the main endpoint of cardiovascular death and MI. Post hoc analysis demonstrated some reductions in other endpoints in subgroups. Further analysis from the FIELD study has shown a significant reduction in microalbuminuria and diabetic retinopathy. The mechanism for this is unknown, and further research is required.

3.4 **Conclusions**

The use of statins is now a routine part of the management of middle-aged and elderly diabetic patients. Serious consideration should be given to using high-dose statins in patients with existing cardiovascular disease, especially following acute coronary syndromes.

Key references

Ahmed S, Cannon CP, Murphy SA, Brunwaold E (2006). Acute coronary syndromes and diabetes: is intensive lipid lowering beneficial? Results of the PROVE IT-TIMI 22 trial. *European Heart Journal*, **27**: 2323–9.

Cholesterol Trialists' (CTT) Collaborators (2008). Efficacy of cholesterol-lowering therapy in 18 686 people with diabetes in 14 randomised trials of statins: a meta-analysis. *Lancet*, **371**: 117–25.

Colhoun HM, Betteridge DJ, Durrington PN, Hitman GA, Neil HA, Livingstone SJ, et al. on behalf of the CARDS investigators (2004). Primary prevention of cardiovascular disease with atorvastatin in type 2 diabetes in the Collaborative Atorvastatin Diabetes Study (CARDS): multicentre randomised placebo-controlled trial. *Lancet*, **364**: 685–96.

Costa J, Borges M, David C, Vaz Carneiro A (2006). Efficacy of lipid lowering drug treatment for diabetic and non-diabetic patients: meta-analysis of randomised controlled trails. *British Medical Journal*, **332**: 1115–24.

Goldberg RB, Mellies MJ, Sacks FM, Move LA, Howard BV, Howard WJ, et al. for the CARE Investigators (1998). Cardiovascular events and their reduction with pravastatin in diabetic and glucose-intolerant myocardial infarction survivors with average cholesterol levels. Subgroup analyses in the Cholesterol And Recurrent Events (CARE) Trial. *Circulation*, **98**: 2513–19.

Heart Protection Study Collaborative Group (2003). MRC/BHF Heart Protection Study of cholesterol-lowering with simvastatin in 5963 people with diabetes: a randomised placebo-controlled trial. *Lancet*, **361**: 2005–16.

Keech A, Colquhoun D, Best J, Kirby A, Simes RJ, Hunt D, *et al.* for the LIPID Study Group (2003). Secondary prevention of cardiovascular events with long-term pravastatin in patients with diabetes or impaired fasting glucose: results from the LIPID trial. *Diabetes Care*, **26**: 2713–21.

Pyorala K, Pedersen TR, Kjekshus J, Faergeman O, Olsson AG, Thorgeirsson G and the Scandinavian Simvastatin Survival Study (4S) Group (1997). Cholesterol lowering with simvastatin improves prognosis of diabetic patients with coronary heart disease. A subgroup analysis of the Scandinavian Simvastatin Survival Study (4S). *Diabetes Care*, **20**: 614–20.

Shepherd J, Barter P, Carmena R, Deedwania P, Fruchart JC, Haffner S, *et al.* for the Treating to New Targets Investigators (2006). Effect of lowering LDL cholesterol substantially below currently recommended levels in patients with coronary heart disease and diabetes: the Treating to New Targets (TNT) study. *Diabetes Care*, **29**: 1220–6.

Chapter 4

Hypertension in diabetes

Miles Fisher

> ### Key points
>
> - Hypertension is common in patients with type 2 diabetes and is a component of the metabolic syndrome.
> - Aggressive treatment of hypertension in patients with type 2 diabetes reduces microvascular complications, strokes, myocardial infarctions (MIs), and total mortality.
> - The greatest benefit is obtained by aggressive lowering of blood pressure, and the choice of antihypertensive drug is a secondary consideration.
> - Older antihypertensive agents may be less effective than newer agents in lowering blood pressure, and angiotensin-converting enzyme inhibitors and angiotensin-II receptor antagonists may have some advantages in further reducing acute events and diabetic nephropathy.
> - Targets for blood pressure lowering are lower in people with diabetes, and to achieve these targets requires the use of multiple antihypertensive drugs.

4.1 Mechanisms of hypertension in diabetes

Hypertension is common in patients with diabetes. In patients with type 1 diabetes, blood pressure is slightly increased compared to age-matched non-diabetic control subjects. Blood pressure increases further in type 1 patients who have microalbuminuria, and hypertension is common in patients with macroalbuminuria (see also Chapter 10).

Hypertension is very common in people with type 2 diabetes, is two–three times more common than in the age-matched general population, and is a component of the metabolic syndrome. Obese people have a greater risk of hypertension. For each unit increase in body mass index the prevalence of hypertension increases by 1.0–1.5%. There are several possible explanations for the link between insulin resistance and hypertension (Box 4.1).

> **Box 4.1 Possible mechanisms of hypertension with insulin resistance**
>
> - Insulin-stimulated sodium and water retention through the distal renal tubules
> - Increased contractility and vascular resistance
> - Increased sympathetic stimulation
> - Vascular smooth muscle proliferation
> - Impaired insulin-mediated vasodilation.

Untreated hypertension in diabetes increases the risk of cardiovascular disease (myocardial infarction (MI), congestive cardiac failure, stroke) and microvascular disease (retinopathy, nephropathy).

If the current definition of hypertension of a blood pressure greater than 140/90mmHg is adopted, then at least 40% of patients with type 2 diabetes will have hypertension. It should be noted that the risk of vascular events in people with diabetes increases even within the normal range, that is, blood pressure is a continuous risk factor. Recent evidence from the Action in Diabetes and Vascular disease: preterAx and diamicroN-MR Controlled Evaluation (ADVANCE) study shows that reduction of blood pressure in diabetic patients with a 'normal' blood pressure, that is, less that 140/90mmHg will reduce events (see Section 4.2.3).

There are several endocrine diseases where diabetes and hypertension are both present, including Cushing's syndrome, phaeochromocytoma, and acromegaly. These are not routinely screened for in hypertensive diabetic patients, and further investigation should be prompted by the presence of other clinical features.

4.1.1 **Investigation of hypertension in diabetic patients**

The measurement of blood pressure is an integral part of diabetes care, and in some clinical areas it is measured at each visit. Blood pressure should be measured following the recommendations of the British Hypertension Society (Box 4.2). Hypertension in diabetes is defined as a systolic blood pressure of 140mmHg or more, and/or a diastolic blood pressure of 90mmHg or more.

Ambulatory blood pressure monitoring (ABPM) or home blood pressure readings are usually lower than clinic readings, and thresholds and targets should be adjusted downwards by 10/5mmHg. They are useful for identifying 'white coat' hypertension and for monitoring the response to treatment.

A diabetic patient with hypertension should have urea and electrolytes checked, with urinalysis for microalbuminuria and proteinuria. An ECG should be performed looking for voltage criteria of left ventricular hypertrophy. If present, this carries a worse prognosis, and may influence the choice of anti-hypertensive drug. Imaging of the kidneys should be performed looking for renal artery stenosis if hypertension proves resistant to treatment.

> **Box 4.2 British Hypertension Society recommendations for the measurement of blood pressure by standard mercury sphygmomanometer or semi-automated device**
>
> - Use a properly maintained, calibrated, and validated device.
> - Measure sitting blood pressure routinely: standing blood pressures should be recorded if there is a suspicion of orthostatic hypotension.
> - Remove tight clothing, support arm at heart level, ensure hand relaxed, and avoid talking during the measurement procedure.
> - Use cuff of appropriate size.
> - Lower mercury column slowly (2mm/s).
> - Read blood pressure to the nearest 2mmHg.
> - Measure diastolic at disappearance of sounds (phase V).
> - Take the mean of at least two readings; more recordings are needed if notable differences between initial measurements are found.
> - Do not treat on the basis of an isolated reading.

4.2 **Evidence of benefit in reducing blood pressure in diabetes**

Patients with diabetes were excluded from many early trials of blood pressure lowering.

4.2.1 **Studies in isolated systolic hypertension**

The first clear evidence that blood pressure lowering was of benefit in people with diabetes was from studies in older patients with isolated systolic hypertension. As the study group was older, many subjects with diabetes were recruited, allowing diabetic subgroup analysis. The Systolic Hypertension in the Elderly Program (SHEP) study examined the use of chlortalidone compared to placebo in systolic hypertension. There was a significant reduction in major cardiovascular events, with a greater absolute risk reduction in the diabetic subgroup. In the Systolic hypertension-Europe (Syst-Eur) study the benefits of nitrendipine compared with placebo were greater in the diabetic subgroup, with significant reductions in cardiovascular events, cardiovascular mortality, and all-cause mortality.

Together these studies demonstrated a significant reduction in cardiovascular events when hypertension was treated in people with diabetes.

4.2.2 **United Kingdom Prospective Diabetes Study**

The United Kingdom Prospective Diabetes Study (UKPDS), described in Chapter 2, was a study of tight blood glucose control in patients with type 2 diabetes. During recruitment to the UKPDS the high prevalence of hypertension was noted, so a blood pressure study was nested within the main study, comparing tight blood pressure control (mean blood pressure 144/82mmHg) with less tight control (mean 154/87mmHg). One-quarter of the total study population was also in the blood pressure study, and this was initially called the Hypertension in Diabetes Study (HDS). Tight control was obtained with a blood-pressure-lowering regimen based on either captopril or atenolol, but many patients required three or more drugs.

Compared to the group with less tight control, tight control of blood pressure reduced both macrovascular and microvascular complications of diabetes (Figure 4.1). No differences were observed when comparing treatment based on captopril, with treatment based on atenolol, but the study was statistically underpowered for this comparison.

4.2.3 **Blood pressure targets in diabetes**

The Hypertension Optimal Treatment (HOT) trial was a larger but shorter study in 18 790 patients. The aim of the study was to compare the benefits of three diastolic blood pressure targets, <90mmHg, <85mmHg, and <80mmHg, on major cardiovascular events (non-fatal myocardial infarction (MI), non-fatal stroke, cardiovascular death). The separation between the groups was less than intended, and the achieved blood pressures were 144/85mmHg, 141/83mmHg, and 140/81mmHg.

In the study, overall there was a reduction in major cardiovascular events comparing the group with a target blood pressure of < 85mmHg compared to a target of <90mmHg, but there was no further benefit with a lower target of <80mmHg. *Post hoc* subgroup analysis of the 1501 diabetic subjects (8%) showed a further significant reduction in major cardiovascular events in diabetic patients allocated to the lower target blood pressure.

When taken together, UKPDS and HOT show that tight control of blood pressure reduced events more than less tight control, and indicate that a target blood pressure of 140/80 is supported by evidence, but that several agents may be required to reach the target.

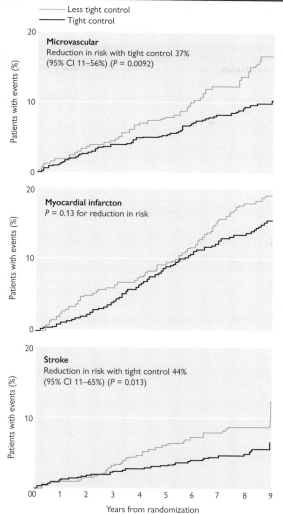

Figure 4.1 UKPDS blood pressure study reductions in micro- and macrovascular endpoints

Less tight control
Tight control

Microvascular
Reduction in risk with tight control 37%
(95% CI 11–56%) (P = 0.0092)

Myocardial infarcton
P = 0.13 for reduction in risk

Stroke
Reduction in risk with tight control 44%
(95% CI 11–65%) (P = 0.013)

Years from randomization

Figure 4.1 is reproduced with permission from UK Prospective Diabetes Study Group (1998). *British Medical Journal*, **317**: 703–13.

The recent ADVANCE study has shown that blood pressure lowering to even lower levels (135/75mmHg), and in patients not deemed to have hypertension at baseline, further reduces cardiovascular events in diabetic patients (Figure. 4.2). The systolic pressure is still higher than the target of <130/80mmHg that is recommended in some guidelines.

Figure 4.2 ADVANCE study reductions in (a) combined primary end point and (b) total mortality

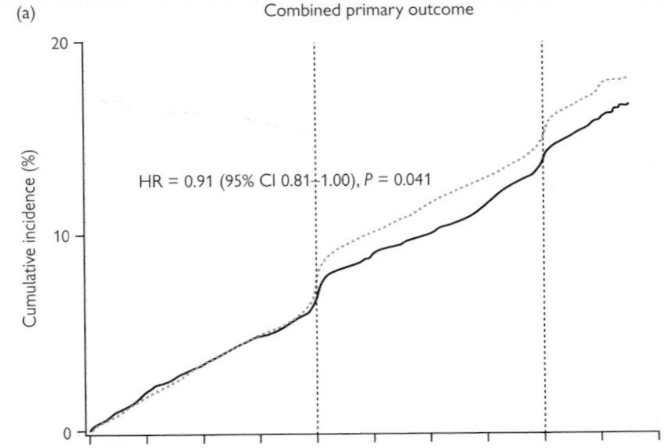
(a)
Combined primary outcome
Cumulative incidence (%)
20
10
0
HR = 0.91 (95% CI 0.81–1.00), P = 0.041

Number at risk

Placebo	5571	5458	5362	5253	5078	4909	4805	4703	4383	1854
Per-Ind	5568	5448	2361	5260	5122	4986	4906	4806	4466	1895

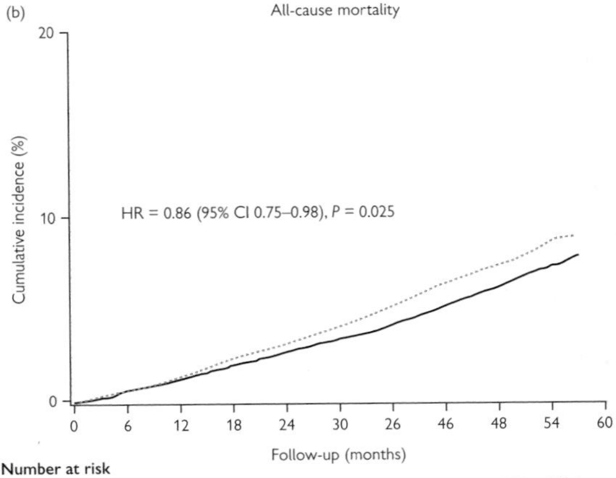
(b)
All-cause mortality
Cumulative incidence (%)
20
10
0
HR = 0.86 (95% CI 0.75–0.98), P = 0.025
0
6
12
18
24
30
26
46
48
54
60
Follow-up (months)

Number at risk

Placebo	5571	5535	5493	5433	5397	5340	5282	5211	4955	2126
Per-Ind	5568	5533	5500	5455	5416	5377	5334	5277	5014	2165

Figure 4.2 is reproduced with permission from ADVANCE Collaborative Group (2007). *Lancet*, **370**: 829–40.

4.3 Which antihypertensive drug to use?

The major benefit is the amount of blood pressure reduction, and many people with diabetes will require multiple agents to reach blood pressure targets, so the question is not 'Which drug to use?' but 'Which drugs to use, and in what combinations?' (Box 4.3). Recent studies have indicated that atenolol is less effective than other therapies in reducing blood pressure in people with diabetes, with a lesser reduction in cardiovascular events, and first-line therapy is usually based on either an ACE inhibitor or angiotensin-II receptor antagonist, with subsequent addition of either a calcium-channel blocker or a diuretic (Figure 4.3).

Box 4.3 Proven anti-hypertensive drugs in diabetes

Angiotensin-converting enzyme inhibitors
- Captopril
- Enalapril
- Fosinopril
- Lisinopril
- Perindopril
- Ramipril
- Trandolapril

Angiotensin-II receptor antagonists
- Irbesartan
- Losartan

Calcium-channel blockers
- Amlodipine
- Nifedipine
- Nitrendipine
- Verapamil

Diuretics
- Chlortalidone
- Co-Amilozide
- Indapamide

Beta-blockers
- Atenolol

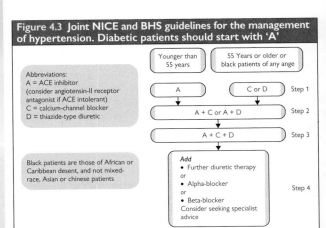

Figure 4.3 Joint NICE and BHS guidelines for the management of hypertension. Diabetic patients should start with 'A'

4.3.1 **Angiotensin-converting enzyme inhibitors**

Angiotensin-converting enzyme inhibitors (ACE inhibitors) inhibit the conversion of angiotensin-I to -II. The main side effects of ACE inhibitors are cough, hypotension, renal impairment, and angioedema. Cough is caused by inhibition of the breakdown of bradykinin, which by improving endothelial function might mediate some of the cardiovascular benefits of ACE inhibitors. ACE inhibitors slightly increase insulin sensitivity, which may improve glycaemic control in patients with diabetes, and provoke hypoglycaemia when used in combination with oral antidiabetic drugs or insulin.

Captopril was demonstrated to reduce microvascular and macrovascular outcomes in the UKPDS blood pressure study. Lisinopril was one of the treatment arms in the Antihypertensive and Lipid-Lowering treatment to prevent Heart Attack Trial (ALLHAT) and perindopril was combined with amlodipine in the Anglo-Scandinavian Cardiac Outcomes (ASCOT) trial. Perindopril was also used as the basis for blood pressure treatment in the Perindopril Protection against Recurrent Stroke Study (PROGRESS) that is described in more detail in Chapter 9.

The recent ADVANCE study examined the use of a fixed dose combination of perindopril and indapamide compared to placebo in 11 140 patients with type 2 diabetes and cardiovascular disease or cardiovascular risk factors.

The potential benefits of ACE inhibitors on renal and cardiac outcomes in patients with diabetic nephropathy are described in Chapter 10.

4.3.2 **Angiotensin-II receptor antagonists**

Angiotensin-II receptor antagonists (ARAs) act highly selectively at angiotensin 1 (AT$_1$) receptors. Unlike ACE inhibitors, ARAs do not inhibit the breakdown of bradykinin, and so are a useful alternative for patients who are unable to tolerate ACE inhibitors because of cough.

Losartan Intervention For Endpoint reduction in hypertension (LIFE) was a trial comparing losartan and atenolol-based therapy in 9193 patients with hypertension and ECG criteria of left ventricular hypertrophy. Losartan significantly reduced the primary composite endpoint of cardiovascular death, MI, and stroke, with significant reductions in stroke, but not MI or cardiovascular death. In 1195 patients with pre-existing diabetes (13%) losartan significantly reduced the composite endpoint and cardiovascular and total mortality, but the reduction in strokes and MI was not significant.

There have been several other publications from the LIFE study that have given useful information about cardiovascular risk in type 2 diabetes (Box 4.4).

The potential benefits of ARAs on renal and cardiac outcomes in patients with diabetic nephropathy are described in Chapter 10.

Box 4.4 Results from the LIFE study

Principal result

- Losartan was more effective than atenolol in reducing the composite of cardiovascular death, myocardial infarction and stroke in hypertensive diabetic patients with ECG criteria of left ventricular hypertrophy.

Other important results

- Losartan was more effective than atenolol in reducing sudden cardiac death in people with diabetes.
- Systolic and diastolic left ventricular function was impaired independent of left ventricular mass, most likely reflecting the adverse effects of diabetes on ventricular function.
- Patients with diabetes had less regression of left ventricular hypertrophy in response to antihypertensive therapy than patients without diabetes.
- Increasing baseline albuminuria related to increased risk for cardiovascular events in patients with diabetes, and benefits of losartan seemed to be greatest in patients with the highest baseline urinary albumin excretion.
- The development of new-onset diabetes (NOD) could be predicted using a score based on baseline serum glucose concentration, body mass index, serum HDL cholesterol, systolic blood pressure, and a history of prior use of antihypertensive drugs.

4.3.3 **Calcium-channel blockers**

Calcium-channel blockers were one of the first classes of drugs to be of proven benefit when used to treat hypertension in diabetes. Nitrendipine was used in the Syst-Eur study, and treatment in the HOT trial was based on felodipine. Amlodipine was used in ALLHAT and ASCOT. Initial concerns that nifedipine might increase MIs in people with diabetes have not been substantiated.

4.3.4 **Diuretics**

Bendroflumethiazide, formerly bendrofluazide, is a thiazide diuretic that is frequently recommended in treatment guidelines, but the evidence for its use in people with diabetes is remarkably slim. It was used in combination with atenolol in the ASCOT study.

Chlortalidone, formerly chlorthalidone, is a thiazide-related compound that reduced events in diabetic patients with systolic hypertension in the SHEP study. It was one of the treatment arms in the ALLHAT study, which compared chlortalidone with lisinopril, amlodipine, and doxazosin. Lisinopril, amlodipine, and chlortalidone were equally effective, but this trial has been strongly criticized because of poor study design.

Indapamide is chemically related to chlortalidone, and is claimed to lower blood pressure with less metabolic disturbance. It was used as an optional part of the treatment in the PROGRESS study, and in fixed combination with perindopril in the ADVANCE study.

4.3.5 **Beta-blockers**

Most of the evidence for the use of beta-blockers in diabetes concerns atenolol. In the UKPDS atenolol was as effective as the ACE-inhibitor captopril in reducing microvascular and macrovascular events, although in retrospect the study was underpowered to show any difference. In the LIFE study, atenolol was inferior to losartan in reducing the primary composite endpoint of cardiovascular death, MI, and stroke.

More recently the ASCOT study compared newer treatments (amlodipine plus perindopril) versus older treatments (atenolol plus bendroflumethiazide) in 19 257 patients with hypertension and cardiovascular risk. A total of 5145 subjects (27%) were known to have diabetes at randomization.

The study was stopped early because of a significant reduction in total mortality comparing newer and older treatments. The reduction in the primary endpoint (non-fatal MI, cardiovascular death) was not statistically significant, but most of the secondary endpoints were significantly reduced.

The study was designed to give equal effectiveness in reducing blood pressure, but in fact the newer treatments were more effective, with a mean blood pressure of 136/78mmHg with newer treatments versus 138/79 with older treatments. When a statistical correction was made for the difference in blood pressures, the newer treatments were still more effective in reducing vascular endpoints.

Because of the results of ASCOT and LIFE, beta-blockers are no longer recommended as first-line anti-hypertensive drugs unless there is another indication for their use such as post-myocardial infarction, chronic heart failure, or the symptomatic treatment of angina.

4.3.6 **Other agents**

Doxazosin is an alpha-blocker. The doxazosin arm of ALLHAT was stopped prematurely, and doxazosin should be reserved for diabetic patients who are unable to tolerate alternatives or have not reached blood pressure targets despite multiple drugs.

4.4 **Risks of diabetes with antihypertensive drugs**

The development of NOD has been a secondary endpoint in several blood pressure and cardiovascular trials. Beta-blockers and diuretics increase the risk of NOD, and calcium-channel blockers are neutral. ACE inhibitors and ARAs seem to reduce the development of NOD in cardiovascular patients and there are several hypothetical explanations for this (Box 4.5). In the Diabetes REduction Assessment with ramipril and rosiglitazone Medication (DREAM) trial ramipril treatment did not significantly effect the progression to diabetes. Regression to normoglycaemia, which was a secondary endpoint, was significantly increased with ramipril.

> Box 4.5 Possible explanations for the reduction in new-onset diabetes with ACE inhibitors and ARAs
>
> **Blockade of adverse effects of angiotensin II**
> - Improved insulin signalling
> - Improved skeletal muscle blood flow
> - Reduced oxidative stress
> - Reduced sympathetic activation
> - Suppressed adipogenesis
> - Increased islet cell blood flow.
>
> **Effects beyond the renin-angiotensin system**
> - Enhanced glucose metabolism by activation of bradykinin/nitric oxide pathways (ACE inhibitors)
> - Improved glucose and lipid metabolism by activation of PPAR gamma.

4.5 **Conclusions**

The management of hypertension in patients with diabetes has been proved to reduce macrovascular and microvascular endpoints. Several drug classes are of proven benefit, and multiple drugs may be required to reach blood pressure targets.

Key references

ADVANCE Collaborative Group (2007). Effects of a fixed combination of perindopril and indapamide on macrovascular and microvascular outcomes in patients with type 2 diabetes mellitus (the ADVANCE trial): a randomised controlled trial. *Lancet*, **370**: 829–40.

ALLHAT Officers and Coordinators for the ALLHAT Collaborative Research Group (2002). Major outcomes in high-risk hypertensive patients randomized to angiotensin-converting enzyme inhibitor or calcium-channel blocker vs diuretic: The Antihypertensive and Lipid-Lowering Treatment to Prevent Heart Attack Trial (ALLHAT). *Journal of American Medical Association*, **288**: 2981–97.

Curb JD, Pressel SL, Cutler JA, Savage PJ, Appelgate WB, Black H, et al. (1996). Effect of diuretic-based antihypertensive treatment on cardiovascular disease risk in older diabetic patients with isolated systolic hypertension. *Journal of American Medical Association*, **276**: 1886–92.

Hansson L, Zanchetti A, Carruthers SG, Dahlof B, Elmfeldt D, Julius S, et al. for the HOT Study Group (1998). Effects of intensive blood-pressure lowering and low-dose aspirin in patients with hypertension: principal results of the Hypertension Optimal Treatment (HOT) randomised trial. *Lancet*, **351**: 1755–62.

Lindholm LH, Ibsen H, Dahlöf B, Devereux RB, Beevers G, de Faire U, et al., for the LIFE study Group (2002). Cardiovascular morbidity and mortality in patients with diabetes in the Losartan Intervention For Endpoint reduction in hypertension study (LIFE): a randomised trial against atenolol. *Lancet*, **359**: 1004–10.

Tuomilehto J, Rastenyte D, Birkenhager WH, Thijs L, Antikainen R, Bulpitt CJ, et al. for the Systolic Hypertension in Europe Trial Investigators (1999). Effects of calcium-channel blockade in older patients with diabetes and systolic hypertension. *New England Journal of Medicine*, **340**: 677–84.

UK Prospective Diabetes Study Group (1998). Tight blood pressure control and risk of macrovascular and microvascular complications in type 2 diabetes: UKPDS 38. *British Medical Journal*, **317**: 703–13.

Chapter 5

Coronary heart disease in diabetes

Adil Rajwani and Stephen Wheatcroft

> **Key points**
>
> - Hyperglycaemia, insulin resistance, oxidative stress, dyslipidaemia, inflammation, and clotting abnormalities are all implicated in increased atherothrombosis in diabetes.
> - Individuals with diabetes have more severe and rapidly progressive coronary artery disease, with greater multi-vessel and left main coronary artery involvement.
> - The proportion of individuals with non-typical symptoms or silent ischaemia is increased in the presence of diabetes.
> - Whether asymptomatic individuals with diabetes should be screened for the presence of cardiovascular disease remains unclear at present.
> - Intensive secondary prevention is essential with antiplatelet, antihypertensive, and lipid-lowering drugs.

5.1 Background

5.1.1 Epidemiology

The epidemiology of cardiovascular disease in diabetes is described in Chapter 1. The risk of death from coronary heart disease (CHD) in individuals with diabetes is two- to threefold greater than in those without diabetes. Women with diabetes are particularly prone to cardiovascular disease. The increased cardiovascular risk attributable to diabetes is only partly explained by concomitant risk factors, including hypertension, obesity, dyslipidaemia, and smoking. This suggests that components of the diabetes phenotype, including hyperglycaemia, insulin resistance, inflammation, endothelial dysfunction, and oxidative stress, are important mediators of the elevated CHD risk and increased mortality.

Although age-adjusted mortality rates for cardiovascular disease in the general population have been declining in recent years, there has been an increase in mortality in patients with diabetes.

5.2 **Pathology**

5.2.1 **Plaque development**

Atherosclerotic plaques develop through a complex process resulting from endothelial cell dysfunction, adhesion and incorporation of inflammatory cells, lipid deposition, smooth muscle cell proliferation, and changes in intercellular matrix. The factors which may contribute to atherosclerosis in diabetes are illustrated in Figure 5.1.

Endothelial cell dysfunction, one of the earliest detectable vascular abnormalities in individuals who subsequently develop atherosclerosis, is a key factor in plaque development and progression. Characterized by an imbalance in the production of pro- and anti-atherosclerotic molecules by endothelial cells, endothelial dysfunction is closely related to insulin resistance and may precede the development of type 2 diabetes by many years. In fact, insulin resistance has emerged as a unifying aetiologic factor linking type 2 diabetes with atherosclerosis.

Hyperglycaemia contributes to atherosclerosis by multiple mechanisms, including increased production of advanced glycation end products (AGE), which favour overproduction of reactive oxygen species. Increased expression of adhesion molecules by endothelial

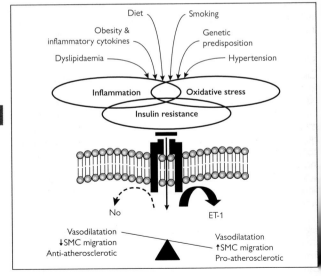

Figure 5.1 Diabetes is associated with multiple abnormalities which induce endothelial dysfunction. This shifts the balance between the production of molecules such as nitric oxide (NO) and endothelin (ET-1), favouring the development of atherosclerosis.

cells and production of pro-inflammatory chemokines and cytokines promote infiltration of macrophages and other inflammatory cells. Diabetes favours uptake of oxidized LDL and stimulates macrophages to form lipid-laden foam cells. Diabetes is also associated with vascular smooth muscle cell proliferation. Apoptosis of inflammatory cells and smooth muscle cells contributes to the formation of the necrotic core. Increased expression of matrix metalloproteinases in diabetes permits plaque remodelling and may favour plaque rupture.

Post-mortem studies comparing hearts from individuals with and without diabetes who have died suddenly confirm a greater total plaque load, with a predisposition to distal coronary artery location and larger necrotic cores, in individuals with diabetes. Plaques from patients with diabetes have greater numbers of macrophages and T lymphocytes, increased expression of receptors for advanced glycation end products, and more smooth muscle cell and macrophage apoptosis.

5.2.2 **Vessel remodelling**

In the early stages of plaque development, the coronary artery typically remodels outward, thereby maintaining a near-normal lumen. In individuals with diabetes, however, both pathological and intra-vascular ultrasound studies demonstrate that the vessel remodels inward. This results in significant luminal compromise by the developing plaque, promoting ischaemic symptoms and favouring coronary occlusion subsequent to plaque rupture.

5.2.3 **Hypercoagulability**

Clinical manifestations of plaque rupture are attributable to the formation of a platelet-rich thrombus. Diabetes is associated with a number of abnormalities promoting platelet aggregation and thrombus formation. Platelets are larger in individuals with diabetes, with greater expression of glycoprotein IIb/IIIa and increased tendency to aggregate as compared to individuals without diabetes. Circulating concentrations of coagulation factors VII, XII, and fibrinogen are increased, as are plasma levels of the fibrinolytic inhibitor, plasminogen activator inhibitor-1. In addition, diabetes has important effects on fibrin structure and function, generating a clot with a denser structure which is more resistant to lysis.

5.3 **Features of coronary disease in diabetes**

5.3.1 **Pathological studies**

Large autopsy studies have demonstrated that severity and extent of coronary artery disease are markedly increased in patients with diabetes. In a recent population-based post-mortem study, high-grade coronary stenoses were found in 75% of men and women with diabetes, in contrast to 55% of those without diabetes. After adjusting for age and sex, the likelihood of a high atherosclerosis burden was equivalent in patients with diabetes without clinical CHD and in patients without diabetes with clinical CHD. The study revealed high prevalence of sub-clinical coronary artery disease in individuals with diabetes without a history of CHD.

Debulking of atherosclerotic plaques by percutaneous coronary intervention with directional coronary atherectomy allows the plaque debris to be exported and examined histologically. Plaque debris from patients with diabetes has a significantly higher macrophage contact than that from individuals without diabetes.

5.3.2 **Angiographic studies**

Angiographic series confirm a greater atherosclerotic burden in patients with diabetes. A recent single-centre study compared the findings of consecutive patients undergoing coronary angiography according to the presence or absence of diabetes. Coronary disease, evaluated objectively with a severity scoring system, was more severe in the patients with diabetes and included higher coronary occlusion rates. In other angiographic studies the presence of diabetes was associated with more diffuse, multi-vessel, left main and distal coronary artery disease with poorer collateral development.

5.3.3 **Intra-vascular ultrasound studies**

Intra-vascular ultrasound allows detailed information on vessel wall and plaque morphology to be gathered at the time of coronary angiography. Diabetes is a strong independent predictor of atheroma volume assessed using this technique. Additionally, data from patients with stable angina reveals that diabetes is associated with more plaque calcification, larger necrotic cores, and a greater prevalence of rupture-prone thin cap fibroatheroma.

5.4 **Investigation**

5.4.1 **Choice of investigation**

Investigation may be carried out to confirm the presence of CHD in patients with suggestive symptoms or to screen for CHD in asymptomatic individuals. Choice of modality is influenced by patient-specific factors, in particular the ability to exercise, and by local availability. Functional imaging (nuclear imaging, stress echocardiography and stress magnetic resonance imaging) detects coronary artery disease indirectly by assessing myocardial ischaemia induced by coronary stenoses, whereas X-ray angiography affords direct visualization of the coronary arteries. Other techniques, such as coronary calcium scoring, are less useful in the diagnosis of coronary artery disease but may have a role in screening and risk stratification.

5.4.2 **Exercise electrocardiography**

Exercise electrocardiography (ECG) is widely used but has a lower diagnostic accuracy than perfusion imaging. An adverse prognosis is indicated by poor exercise capacity, exercise-induced ST-segment depression, chronotropic incompetence, or a fall in systolic blood pressure. Sensitivity of exercise ECG is reduced if the patient is unable to achieve 85% of maximal predicted heart rate response to stress. Up to half of patients with diabetes may be unable to achieve this. Other limitations of exercise electrocardiography include respiratory, neurological, or orthopaedic conditions which preclude exercise and resting ECG abnormalities (e.g. left bundle branch block, left ventricular hypertrophy, ventricular pacing or digoxin use) which prevent interpretation of ST-segment changes with stress.

5.4.1 **Nuclear myocardial perfusion imaging**

The diagnostic utility of single-photon emission computed tomography (SPECT) imaging with pharmacological stress has been extensively demonstrated in the general population, although studies specifically in individuals with diabetes are scarce. The presence of perfusion abnormalities is strongly predictive of subsequent cardiac death and non-fatal myocardial infarction in both symptomatic and asymptomatic populations with diabetes. Clinical outcomes are directly related to the severity and size of the perfusion abnormalities. A 'normal' SPECT scan has a lower negative predictive value for future cardiovascular events in patients with diabetes than in the general population. This may reflect the more rapid progression of atherosclerosis in patients with diabetes.

5.4.2 **Stress echocardiography**

Stress echocardiography assesses regional myocardial wall motion in response to exercise or, more usually, pharmacological stress. In unselected populations, stress echocardiography has similar sensitivity and specificity for detection of coronary artery disease to SPECT imaging. Small-scale studies in individuals with diabetes support a similar sensitivity and specificity to non-diabetic individuals. Several studies have confirmed that stress-induced wall motion abnormalities predict cardiovascular death and non-fatal myocardial infarction in patients with diabetes. Similar to the SPECT imaging, the severity of echocardiographic abnormalities predict long-term prognosis and the negative predictive value of stress echocardiography is diminished in individuals with diabetes.

5.4.3 **Cardiac magnetic resonance imaging**

Cardiac magnetic resonance imaging (MRI) allows comprehensive assessment of myocardial perfusion, viability, coronary anatomy, and global and regional ventricular function in a single study. The high spatial resolution of MRI allows even small perfusion defects to be detected and permits differentiation between subendocardial and transmural infarction. Sensitivity and specificity of cardiac MRI for detection of coronary artery disease in the general population are high but specific studies in patients with diabetes are not available.

5.4.4 **Coronary artery calcium scoring**

Electron-beam computed tomography (EBCT) and multi-slice computed tomography (MSCT) allow non-invasive detection and quantification of coronary artery calcification. Coronary calcium scores are closely correlated with total atherosclerotic burden and the risk of future cardiovascular events, but do not predict the severity of coronary stenoses or provide anatomical information. In the general population, the coronary calcium score may provide incremental prognostic information over conventional risk stratification, particularly in individuals at 'intermediate' risk. Limited data are available on coronary artery calcium scoring in individuals with diabetes, although recent studies support the calcium score as an important predictor of mortality, with a greater increase in mortality rate attributable to incremental increases in calcium score in subjects with diabetes than in those without.

5.4.5 **X-ray coronary angiography**

Coronary angiography remains the definitive investigation for the evaluation of coronary artery disease and provides anatomical information on the extent and distribution of disease which is essential for planning subsequent revascularization. There is a small, but not insignificant, incidence of severe complications (death, myocardial infarction or stroke), at approximately 0.1–0.2%. The occurrence of contrast-induced nephropathy is significantly greater in individuals with diabetes (particularly in patients with pre-existing renal impairment) and meticulous attention to pre-hydration should be made wherever possible.

5.4.6 Non-invasive coronary angiography

Recent technical developments in cardiac MRI and MSCT have allowed both techniques to be proposed as alternatives to X-ray angiography. The high spatial resolution and fast scan times of MSCT are particularly attractive for non-invasive angiography. In the general population, the sensitivity and specificity to detect coronary artery disease by MSCT are good, but the increased prevalence of coronary calcification may limit the utility of this modality in populations with diabetes.

5.5 Presentation

5.1 Symptoms of coronary heart disease

HD frequently presents without typical symptoms in individuals with diabetes. The prevalence of 'silent ischaemia' is much higher in those with diabetes than in the general population. Almost one-third of myocardial infarctions in patients with diabetes are not accompanied by chest pain. This may reflect underlying autonomic dysfunction or differences in pain sensitivity associated with diabetes. Similarly, easy fatigability, atypical thoracic discomfort, or effort-related dyspnoea may be the only indications of stable coronary artery disease in patients with diabetes.

5.2 Silent ischaemia

The true prevalence of coronary artery disease in asymptomatic individuals with diabetes is not known. Estimates vary between studies, depending on the imaging modality, study selection criteria, and background risk of the population. The prevalence of coronary atherosclerosis, evaluated using EBCT-derived calcium score, was 6% in a study of over 500 asymptomatic patients with diabetes. Several studies have evaluated silent ischemia, using nuclear imaging or stress echocardiography.

In the Detection of Silent Myocardial Ischaemic in Asymptomatic Diabetics (DIAD) study, the prevalence of abnormal SPECT scans in 22 asymptomatic patients with diabetes and two or more risk factors was 21%. Conventional risk factors did not predict perfusion defects on SPECT. Other studies using SPECT or stress echocardiography suggest a higher prevalence of silent ischaemia (see Table 5.1). All studies in which subsequent clinical events were evaluated confirm a substantially higher risk of cardiovascular death or myocardial infarction in patients with evidence of atherosclerosis or silent ischaemia.

57

Table 5.1 Prevalence of atherosclerosis or silent ischaemia in asymptomatic individuals with diabetes

Study (year of publication)	Participants	Modality	Prevalence of abnormal study (%)
Anand et al. (2006)	510	EBCT	46
Sconamiglio et al. (2006)	1899	Stress Echo	60
Wackers et al. (2004)	522	SPECT	21
Miller et al. (2004)	1738	SPECT	59
Zellweger et al. (2004)	1737	SPECT	39
Rajagopalan et al. (2005)	1427	SPECT	58

5.6 **Screening**

The high prevalence of atherosclerosis and silent ischaemia has prompted some authors and organizations to recommend screening for coronary artery disease in asymptomatic individuals with diabetes. However, this approach is controversial and is not supported by the current evidence base. Studies using SPECT imaging or stress echocardiography suggest that selecting patients with diabetes for screening on the basis of established risk factors would fail to identify a large proportion of individuals with asymptomatic coronary artery disease. In addition, although it is likely that high-risk asymptomatic individuals identified by screening would be targeted for intensive medical therapy or revascularization, whether these manoeuvres result in improved clinical outcomes has not yet been determined. This issue will be addressed, in part, by the forthcoming Bypass Angioplasty Revascularization Investigation 2 Diabetes (BARI 2-D) study. Until such information is available, a pragmatic approach may be to treat established diabetes as a 'cardiovascular risk equivalent' and target all individuals with diabetes with intensive medical therapy and lifestyle advice. A recent consensus statement from the American Diabetes Association suggests that screening, perhaps with cardiac CT, should be reserved for those in whom medical treatment goals cannot be met and in individuals in whom there is strong clinical suspicion of very high-risk coronary artery disease.

5.7 **Symptomatic treatment**

Antianginal drugs improve symptoms by redressing the imbalance between myocardial perfusion and oxygen demand.

5.7.1 **Beta-blockers**

These improve symptom frequency and severity by reducing myocardial oxygen demand. Slowing of resting and exercise-induced heart rate is important in their mode of action. Beta-blockers are effective antianginal drugs which are generally recommended as first-line therapy in patients with or without diabetes.

5.7.2 **Nitrates**

Nitrates are vasodilators which increase subendocardial perfusion by reducing preload (and thus left ventricular end-diastolic pressures and wall-stress) and promoting coronary and collateral dilatation. A nitrate free period is required with long-acting agents to avoid tolerance. Short-acting sub-lingual or buccal nitrates provide rapid symptom relief and can be used prophylactically.

5.7.3 Calcium-channel blockers

Inhibition of calcium influx in vascular smooth muscle cells promotes relaxation, thereby increasing coronary blood flow and systemic vasodilatation. Diltiazem and verapamil have negative chronotropic properties and are useful alternatives to beta-blockers.

5.7.4 Other antianginal drugs

Nicorandil has nitrate-like properties and also vasodilates by opening potassium channels. It is an effective antianginal and reduces the risk of cardiovascular events during follow-up in a randomized trial of patients with stable coronary artery disease. The protective effect was consistent in the subgroup with diabetes, although the trial excluded patients with diabetes who were receiving a sulphonylurea. Ivabradine improves anginal symptoms by limiting heart rate through direct effects on the sinus node, and may be considered in beta-blocker intolerant individuals.

5.8 Secondary prevention

5.8.1 Antiplatelet drugs

Aspirin is recommended in all patients with coronary artery disease, although it is recognized that its efficacy may be diminished in those with diabetes. In a recent large meta-analysis, treatment with aspirin conferred a 22% reduction in vascular events overall, whilst in the subgroup with diabetes, the 7% relative risk reduction did not reach statistical significance. A post hoc analysis of the subgroup with diabetes in the Clopidogrel versus Aspirin in Patients at Risk of Ischemic Events (CAPRIE) study found that clopidogrel reduced the risk of death, myocardial infarction, stroke, or hospital admission compared with aspirin in patients with a history of atherothrombosis. Antiplatelet therapy in acute coronary syndromes is discussed in Chapter 6.

5.8.2 Beta-blockers

Beta-blockers reduce mortality following myocardial infarction and improve symptoms and mortality in patients with heart failure. Beta-blockers are particularly effective in reducing post-infarction mortality in patients with diabetes and are recommended in all patients with coronary artery disease who have experienced an ischaemic event.

5.8.3 Angiotensin-converting enzyme inhibitors

Angiotensin-converting enzyme (ACE) inhibitors improve symptoms and mortality in patients with left ventricular systolic dysfunction and prior MI. The effect is consistent in patients with and without diabetes. ACE inhibitors also improve outcomes in patients with preserved left ventricular function, diabetes, and cardiovascular disease. Ramipril reduced cardiovascular events in patients with diabetes and a previous cardiovascular event or at least one risk factor in the Microalbuminuria Cardiovascular and Renal Outcomes-Heart Outcomes Prevention Evaluation (MICRO-HOPE) substudy. A similar risk reduction was conferred by perindopril in the diabetes subgroup of the EURopean trial On reduction of cardiac events with Perindopril in stable coronary Artery disease (EUROPA). In the Prevention of Events with Angiotensin-Converting Enzyme inhibition (PEACE) study, however trandolapril did not reduce the risk of cardiovascular events in patients with established CHD. This may reflect a lower risk study population and sub-optimal dosing. Meta-analysis of available trials strongly support the use of ACE inhibitors in all patients with diabetes and CHD.

Recently, the Ongoing Telmisartan Alone and in Combination with Ramipril Global Endpoint Trial (ONTARGET) has shown similar cardiovascular benefit to ramipril with the angiotensin-II receptor antagonist telmisartan in patients with vascular disease or high-risk diabetes.

5.8.4 **Lipid-lowering drugs**

The appropriate use of lipid-lowering drugs in individuals with diabetes is discussed in Chapter 3.

5.9 **Conclusions**

CHD is the commonest cause of death in patients with diabetes. Although individuals with diabetes and cardiovascular disease benefit from secondary preventive strategies to similar, if not greater, extent than their counterparts without diabetes, they remain at substantially higher absolute risk of morbidity and mortality. Further research is warranted to more fully understand and resolve this 'residual risk' attributable to diabetes.

Key references

Bax JJ, Inzucchi S E, Bonow R O, Schuijf J D, Freeman M R, Barrett EJ (2007). Cardiac imaging for risk stratification in diabetes, *Diabetes Care*, **30**: 1295–304.

Bax JJ, Young LH, Frye RL, Bonow RO, Steinberg HO, Barrett EJ (2007). Screening for coronary artery disease in patients with diabetes. *Diabetes Care*, **30**: 2729–36.

Fox K, Garcia MA, Ardissino D, Buszman P, Camici PG, Crea F, et al. (2006). Guidelines on the management of stable angina pectoris: executive summary: the Task Force on the Management of Stable Angina Pectoris of the European Society of Cardiology. *European Heart Journal*, **27**: 1341–81.

Haffner SM, Lehto S, Ronnemaa T, Pyorala K, Laakso M (1998). Mortality from coronary heart disease in subjects with type 2 diabetes and in nondiabetic subjects with and without prior myocardial infarction. *New England Journal of Medicine*, **339**: 229–34.

Heart Outcomes Prevention Evaluation Study Investigators (2000). Effects of ramipril on cardiovascular and microvascular outcomes in people with diabetes mellitus: results of the HOPE study and MICRO-HOPE substudy. *Lancet*, **355**: 253–9.

Ryden L, Standl E, Bartnik M, Van den Berge G, Betteridge J, de Boer MJ, et al. (2007). Guidelines on diabetes, pre-diabetes, and cardiovascular diseases: executive summary. The Task Force on Diabetes and Cardiovascular Diseases of the European Society of Cardiology (ESC) and of the European Association for the Study of Diabetes (EASD). *European Heart Journal*, **28**: 88–136.

Wackers FJ, Young LH, Inzucchi SE, Chyun DA, Davey JA, Barrett EJ, et al. (2004). Detection of silent myocardial ischemia in asymptomatic diabetic subjects: the DIAD study. *Diabetes Care*, **27**: 1954–61.

Chapter 6

Acute coronary syndromes in diabetes

Matthew Kahn and Stephen Wheatcroft

Key points

- Individuals with diabetes have an increased incidence of acute coronary syndromes (ACS) and experience poorer outcomes compared with those without diabetes.
- Despite data suggesting that patients with diabetes derive greater benefit from evidence-based therapies for ACS than those without diabetes, these patients less commonly receive treatment according to established guidelines (particularly insulin-treated patients).
- Appropriate management of ACS in patients with diabetes mandates prompt treatment with anti-thrombotic and anti-ischaemic medication, early access to effective reperfusion and revascularization, and institution of optimal secondary preventive measures.

6.1 Clinical features

6.1.1 Epidemiology

The presence of diabetes is common in patients presenting with acute coronary syndromes (ACSs). Around 20–25% of patients with ACS are reported to have diabetes in multi-national registries. In addition, a substantial proportion of patients with ACS who are not known to have diabetes have will have abnormalities when challenged with an oral glucose tolerance test. Overall, 65% of patients presenting with acute myocardial infarction (MI) have demonstrable evidence of impaired glucoregulation.

6.1.2 Pathogenesis

Acute coronary syndromes arise as a consequence of an athero-thrombotic process, typically initiated by spontaneous rupture or erosion of an atherosclerotic coronary plaque. Exposure of the plaque constituents to circulating blood promotes platelet aggregation and thrombosis. Myocardial ischaemia results from thrombotic occlusion of the vessel, or from distal embolization of sub-occlusive thrombus compounded by vasospasm.

A number of factors predispose individuals with diabetes to plaque rupture, as illustrated in Figure 6.1. Insulin resistance, oxidative stress, and hyperglycaemia are associated with endothelial dysfunction—a key feature in the development and progression of atherosclerosis.

The presence of diabetes is also linked with increased vascular inflammation, characterized by greater lymphocytic infiltration, increased production of pro-inflammatory cytokines, and upregulation of matrix metalloproteinases which predispose the plaque to rupture. Diabetes is also associated with a pro-thrombotic state. Platelets are larger with an increased propensity to adhere to the vessel wall. A greater concentration of cell surface glycoprotein IIb/IIIa receptors facilitates aggregation upon stimulation. Altered clotting factors and reduced concentrations of endogenous fibrinolytic mediators in individuals with diabetes are complicit in increasing the likelihood of a plaque rupture resulting in thrombotic complications and the clinical manifestation of an ACS.

6.1.2 **Influence of diabetes on clinical outcomes**

Despite implementation of contemporary evidence-based therapies, diabetes confers an adverse prognosis for patients presenting with ACS. Both short-term outcomes and long-term survival are substantially impaired in individuals with diabetes following ACS.

Diabetes increases the risk of a range of complications following ACS, including left ventricular dysfunction, symptomatic heart failure, recurrent myocardial ischaemia, requirement for urgent revascularization, cardiogenic shock, arrhythmias, re-infarction, stroke, and death.

Figure 6.1 Factors promoting atherosclerosis and plaque rupture in individuals with diabetes

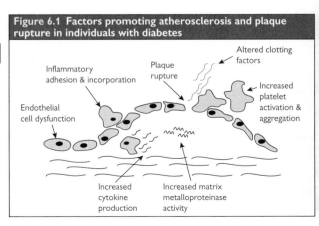

The risk of adverse events is greater in insulin-treated patients with diabetes than in those treated with oral antidiabetic drugs or diet alone.

In the large multi-national Global Registry of Acute Coronary Events (GRACE), which assessed outcomes in over 16 000 patients with ACS, approximately 1 in 4 patients studied had diabetes. The patients with diabetes were less likely to receive effective therapies and were at increased risk of heart failure, renal failure, cardiogenic shock, and death. These differences remained after adjustment for potentially confounding factors. Further observations from GRACE revealed that mortality at 30 days and 1 year was significantly higher amongst patients with diabetes than those without diabetes presenting with ACS.

6.1.3 Classification of ACS

Acute coronary syndromes, in individuals with compatible symptoms, are classified on the basis of the index electrocardiogram (see Table 6.1). ST-segment elevation usually signifies the presence of an occlusive thrombus and mandates emergency reperfusion (by mechanical or pharmacological means) in order to salvage the myocardium under jeopardy. Ischaemic symptoms without ST-segment elevation usually reflect sub-occlusive thrombus. Patients presenting in this manner are typically treated with intensive anti-thrombotic and anti-ischaemic medication, before being considered for urgent coronary angiography and revascularization, if appropriate, following risk stratification. MI is diagnosed on the basis of clinical symptoms, elevation of biomarkers of cardiomyocyte necrosis, or electrocardiographic changes.

Table 6.1 Classification and management of acute coronary syndromes		
	ST-segment elevation (STE-ACS)	**Non-ST-segment elevation (NSTE-ACS)**
Typical ECG changes	ST-segment elevation (or new left bundle-branch block)	ST-segment depression, T-wave inversion, may be normal.
Typical pathology	Plaque rupture → occlusive thrombus	Plaque rupture → non-occlusive thrombus
Immediate management	Reperfusion to limit myocardial necrosis with primary percutaneous coronary intervention if available, or Fibrinolysis	Intensive medical therapy with anti-platelet, anti-thrombotic and anti-ischaemic agents.
Early management	Monitoring on coronary care unit.	Coronary angiography and revascularization if appropriate.
Longer term management	Life-style measures, anti-platelet drugs, beta-blockers, angiotensin-converting enzyme inhibitors, lipid-lowering drugs, cardiac rehabilitation programme.	

6.3 **Non-ST-segment elevation ACSs**

6.3.1 **Anti-platelet therapy**

Platelet activation and aggregation, which play a key role in mediating the clinical features of ACS following rupture of an atherosclerotic plaque, are exaggerated in the presence of diabetes. Intensive anti-platelet therapy is, therefore, a crucial component of the therapeutic approach to ACS.

The benefit of aspirin in athero-thrombotic disease is well established. Although questions remain over the efficacy of aspirin in the primary prevention of cardiovascular disease in diabetes, its use in the acute setting remains universal.

The thienopyridine drugs (e.g. ticlopidine, clopidogrel, and prasugrel) inhibit platelet aggregation in a synergistic manner to aspirin by blocking adenosine diphosphate receptor–dependent platelet activation. The pivotal Clopidogrel in Unstable Angina to Prevent Recurrent Events (CURE) study examined whether the addition of clopidogrel to aspirin in the context of non-ST-segment elevation ACS improved outcome. The addition of clopidogrel to aspirin resulted in a 20% reduction in the composite endpoint of cardiovascular death, MI, or stroke after 12 months of follow-up. The 2840 participants with diabetes had a higher overall vascular event rate than their counterparts without diabetes. The event rate was reduced to a similar extent by the addition of clopidogrel in this group, although this did not reach statistical significance.

Platelets from individuals with diabetes have increased numbers of glycoprotein IIb/IIIa receptors, which constitute the final common pathway for platelet activation when they bind with fibrinogen.

A consistent benefit of IIb/IIIa receptor antagonists in reducing ischaemic complications of non-ST-segment elevation ACS has been demonstrated in multiple trials. In a recent meta-analysis of trials evaluating the use of IIb/IIIa inhibitors in individuals with and without diabetes presenting with ACS, patients with diabetes not only had a reduction in ischaemic complications but a lower mortality. There was no such survival benefit in the group without diabetes. The decrease in mortality was predominantly among those patients with diabetes who underwent percutaneous coronary intervention.

6.3.2 **Anti-ischaemic therapy**

Beta-blockers are the preferred anti-ischemic drugs in acute coronary syndromes. Although data supporting a mortality benefit in patients with diabetes derive from sub-group analyses of patents with ST-segment elevation MI, published guidelines recommend commencing beta-blockers in all patients with ACS in the absence of contraindications. Beta-blockers are generally well tolerated by patients with diabetes and coronary heart disease.

In addition (or as an alternative) to beta-blockers, nitrates, calcium channel blockers, and nicorandil provide effective relief from ischaemic symptoms, although they have not been shown to result in survival benefits in ACSs.

6.3.3 **Anti-thrombotic therapy**

Unfractionated heparin (UFH) reduces the risk of death and MI in patients with non-ST-segment elevation ACS. Low molecular weight heparins (LMWH) eliminate the need for haematological monitoring and offer the advantage of simpler administration via the subcutaneous route. The LMWH enoxaparin has shown superiority over UFH in the reduction of ischaemic events in clinical trials although it has not been studied exclusively in patients with diabetes.

6.3.4 **Revascularization**

Patients with ACS and diabetes are at high risk for subsequent complications. Several randomized trails have compared medical therapy with an early invasive strategy (comprising coronary angiography and in-patient revascularization when appropriate) in patients presenting with non ST-segment elevation ACS. Pooled data from these studies demonstrate clinical benefit from an early invasive strategy, particularly in patients with moderate- or high-risk features. The magnitude of benefit is similar in patients with and without diabetes. However, as patients with diabetes are at higher absolute risk of adverse events, an early invasive approach confers a greater benefit in this group. The relative merits of percutaneous coronary intervention and coronary artery bypass grafting are discussed in Chapter 7.

6.4 **ST-segment elevation ACSs**

6.4.1 **Initial treatment**

In patients with ST-segment elevation MI, the presence of diabetes is associated with a greater risk of complications and higher short- and long-term mortality. Patients with diabetes present later, are more likely to have atypical symptoms, and more likely to present with cardiogenic shock than patients without diabetes. Despite the higher risk of adverse outcomes, individuals with diabetes are less likely to receive treatment according to established guidelines, particularly pharmacological reperfusion or mechanical reperfusion with percutaneous coronary intervention.

Aspirin produces a rapid anti-thrombotic effect by inhibiting production of thromboxane A2. In unselected patients with ST-segment elevation MI, aspirin alone reduces mortality and confers additional benefit when given in combination with fibrinolytic agents.

Two recent randomized controlled trials have demonstrated additional benefits of clopidogrel when added to aspirin in patients with ST-segment MI receiving fibrinolysis. The addition of clopidogrel improved infarct-related vessel patency, reduced re-infarction, and improved mortality.

Dual oral antiplatelet therapy, with aspirin and a thienopyridine, is mandatory when percutaneous coronary intervention is chosen as the preferred reperfusion strategy.

6.4.2 **Fibrinolysis**

The initial goal in the management of ST-segment elevation MI is to achieve reperfusion of the infarction-related artery and limit infarction size. The Fibrinolytic Therapy Trialists Collaborative group reviewed early adverse outcomes and mortality in nine large randomized trials of fibrinolytic therapy in 58 600 patients with suspected ST-segment elevation MI. Mortality was reduced from 11.5% in the control group to 9.6% in patients receiving fibrinolysis. Although absolute mortality was higher in the 4529 patients with diabetes, fibrinolysis conferred a greater reduction in mortality in this group (17.3% vs 13.6%).

Despite the clear mortality benefits, registry data demonstrate that patients with diabetes are less likely to receive fibrinolytic therapy than patients without diabetes. Atypical or late presentation to medical care, or unfounded concerns over haemorrhagic complications of fibrinolysis in patients with diabetes may contribute to this discrepancy.

6.4.3 **Primary percutaneous coronary intervention**

Primary percutaneous coronary intervention (PCI) for ST-segment elevation MI yields more favourable outcomes than fibrinolytic therapy, with pooled analysis from randomized trials demonstrating significant reductions in all-cause mortality, non-fatal re-infarction, and stroke. A recent analysis of individual patient data from 19 trials of primary PCI versus fibrinolysis compared outcomes in patients with and without diabetes. Absolute 30-day mortality was higher in patients with diabetes. However, primary PCI was associated with similar reductions in mortality compared with fibrinolysis in patients with diabetes (relative risk reduction 51%) and those without diabetes (relative risk reduction 41%).

Primary PCI is now recommended as the preferred reperfusion strategy for ST-segment elevation MI, provided it can be delivered promptly by centres with experience in the technique.

6.4.4 **Early post-infarction management**

Treatment with beta-blockers reduces mortality in unselected patients following MI. Sub-group analyses from randomized controlled trials demonstrate that beta-blockers are particularly effective in reducing mortality and recurrent MI in patients with diabetes. In the absence of contraindications, oral beta-blockers are recommended for all patients with diabetes following MI. Angiotensin-converting enzyme inhibitors started in unselected patients within 24 hours of an ST-segment MI reduce mortality and the risk of developing heart failure. The benefits are similar in patients with and without diabetes. Greater benefits are apparent in those with symptoms of heart failure or evidence of left ventricular systolic dysfunction. The angiotensin-II receptor antagonist valsartan has been associated with an equivalent survival advantage to the angiotensin-converting enzyme inhibitor captopril in high-risk post-infarction patients with diabetes. In patients with heart failure post-MI, the addition of the aldosterone antagonist eplerenone reduces all cause mortality, cardiac mortality, and re-hospitalization. These beneficial effects are consistent in patients with diabetes. However, the potential to induce hyperkalaemia may limit the use of eplerenone in patients with diabetes and microalbuminuria.

6.5 **Management after ACSs**

6.5.1 **Glycaemic control**

Random blood glucose levels in unselected patients admitted with ACS are strongly correlated with adverse short- and long-term outcomes. In patients with diabetes and ACS, high blood glucose levels are highly predictive of in-hospital and subsequent mortality. In the first Diabetes Mellitus Insulin-Glucose Infusion in Acute Myocardial Infarction (DIGAMI) study, patients presenting with ACS and acute hyperglycaemia on admission were randomized to insulin-glucose infusion followed by subcutaneous insulin treatment or to conventional care. Mean blood glucose concentrations were 9.5mmol/L in the intensive insulin-treated group and 11.6mmol/L in the conventional treatment group. Mortality was reduced by 25% after 3.4 years of follow-up in the intensive treatment group. In the DIGAMI-2 study, 1253 patients with type 2 diabetes and ACS were randomized to one of three treatment strategies: insulin-glucose infusion followed by long-term insulin-based glucose control, insulin-glucose infusion followed by standard glucose control, and, routine management of blood glucose according to local practice. The study confirmed that glycaemic control is highly predictive of 2-year mortality but did not reveal any significant difference in outcomes between the three strategies of glycaemic control. However, these results must be interpreted in the context that fasting glucose levels in the first group did not reach target and no difference in long-term glycaemic control, assessed by HbA1c, was achieved between the three groups.

On balance, the strong epidemiological relationship between glucose levels and mortality in patients with co-existing diabetes and coronary heart disease and the mortality reduction demonstrated in the first

DIGAMI study provide compelling arguments for intensive glucose control in patients admitted with ACS.

6.5.2 **Secondary prevention after ACS**

The high risk of recurrent events and increased mortality in patients with diabetes following ACS mandates an intensive approach to secondary prevention.

Although evidence suggests that aspirin may induce less effective platelet inhibition in individuals with diabetes, meta-analysis of secondary prevention trials confirms a consistent protective effect in sub-groups with diabetes. The addition of clopidogrel for up to 12 months following ACS further reduces ischaemic complications and mortality.

Beta-blockers are effective in reducing re-infarction and sudden death in patients with diabetes after MI. Concerns over deterioration in glycaemic control or blunted counter-regulatory responses to hypoglycaemia rarely translate into clinically relevant problems.

Optimal secondary prevention also comprises intensive control of blood pressure and lipid profile, inhibition of the renin-angiotensin-aldosterone system and appropriate lifestyle measures including weight loss and smoking cessation. The roles of statins, angiotensin-converting enzyme inhibitors and angiotensin-II receptor antagonists in secondary prevention in patients with diabetes and cardiovascular disease are discussed elsewhere in this book.

Unfortunately, despite the convincing evidence that secondary preventive measures reduce mortality in patients with coronary heart disease, most therapies are underutilized in patients with diabetes.

6.5.3 **Cardiac rehabilitation**

Cardiac rehabilitation is an important component of comprehensive care for patients following MI. Rehabilitation programmes typically comprise exercise training, education, and behavioural interventions. Their aim is to limit the physical and psychological effects of cardiac disease, reduce the risk of recurrent events, and enhance the psychological and vocational status of participants. Cardiac rehabilitation programmes have been demonstrated to reduce all-cause mortality and improve symptoms, exercise capacity, well-being, lipid profiles, and smoking cessation. The beneficial effects are consistent in participants with and without diabetes. The inclusion of diabetes-focussed multi-factorial interventions in a cardiac rehabilitation programme has recently been shown to lead to greater improvements in cardiovascular risk factors and glycaemic control.

6.6 **Conclusions**

Current data indicate that diabetes is common in patients presenting with ACS, confers a higher risk of mortality and recurrent cardiovascular events, and is associated with a lower likelihood of receiving evidence-based therapies. Although advances in pharmacological and mechanical therapies have improved survival in patients with diabetes and ACS, outcomes remain impaired compared with individuals without diabetes.

Key references

Antithrombotic Trialists' Collaboration (2002). Collaborative meta-analysis of randomised trials of antiplatelet therapy for prevention of death, myocardial infarction, and stroke in high risk patients. *British Medical Journal*, **324**: 71–86.

Malmberg K, Rydén L, Efendic S, Herlitz J, Nicol P, Waldenström A, et al. (1995). Randomized trial of insulin-glucose infusion followed by subcutaneous insulin treatment in diabetic patients with acute myocardial infarction (DIGAMI study): effects on mortality at 1 year. *Journal of American College of Cardiology*, **26**: 57–65.

Malmberg K, Rydén L, Wedel H, Birkeland K, Bootsma A, Dickstein K, et al. (2005). Intense metabolic control by means of insulin in patients with diabetes mellitus and acute myocardial infarction (DIGAMI 2): effects on mortality and morbidity. *European Heart Journal,* **26**: 650–61.

Rydén L, Standl E, Bartnik M, Van den Berghe G, Betteridge J, de Boer MJ, et al. (2007). Guidelines on diabetes, pre-diabetes, and cardiovascular diseases: executive summary. The Task Force on Diabetes and Cardiovascular Diseases of the European Society of Cardiology (ESC) and of the European Association for the Study of Diabetes (EASD). *European Heart Journal*, **28**: 88–136.

Timmer JR, Ottervanger JP, de Boer MJ, Boersma E, Grines CL, et al. Primary Coronary Angioplasty vs Thrombolysis-2 Trialists Collaborators Group (2007). Primary percutaneous coronary intervention compared with fibrinolysis for myocardial infarction in diabetes mellitus: results from the Primary Coronary Angioplasty vs Thrombolysis-2 trial. *Archives of International Medicine,* **167**: 1353–9.

Yusuf S, Zhao F, Mehta SR, Chrolavicius S, Tognoni G, Fox KK, Clopidogrel in Unstable Angina to Prevent Recurrent Events Trial Investigators (2001). Effects of clopidogrel in addition to aspirin in patients with acute coronary syndromes without ST-segment elevation. *New England Journal of Medicine*, **345**: 494–502.

Chapter 7

Coronary revascularization in the patient with diabetes

Stephen Wheatcroft

Key points

- Patients with diabetes represent a substantial proportion of patients undergoing coronary artery bypass graft (CABG) surgery and percutaneous coronary intervention (PCI).

- The diffuse and rapidly progressive nature of coronary disease in individuals with diabetes poses significant challenges for revascularization.

- Despite recent technological advances in surgical and percutaneous techniques, clinical outcomes remain poorer for patients with diabetes compared to those without.

- Selection of revascularization strategy should be based on consideration of the severity and extent of coronary artery disease and the potential for complete revascularization.

- CABG is more effective than PCI in individuals with diabetes and multivessel disease, although the results of large ongoing randomized trials of drug-eluting stents in this setting are awaited.

7.1 Introduction

Individuals with diabetes have a greater prevalence of coronary atherosclerosis, with more diffuse disease, greater left-main stem and multivessel involvement, and accelerated disease progression compared to those without diabetes. Patients with diabetes represent a significant proportion of those requiring coronary revascularization and present specific challenges for both coronary artery bypass graft

(CABG) surgery and percutaneous coronary intervention (PCI). Despite substantial improvements in both surgical and percutaneous techniques over the last decade, the outcomes of revascularization in patients with diabetes remain suboptimal compared with individuals without diabetes.

7.2 Coronary artery bypass grafting

7.2.1 CABG in patients with diabetes

Individuals with diabetes represent up to a quarter of those undergoing CABG surgery. These individuals are often more unwell, older, and have a higher prevalence of hypertension and heart failure than comparable patients without diabetes undergoing CABG. The surgical approach, which usually affords complete revascularization, is particularly appropriate in those with diabetes and multivessel involvement and/or left main-stem disease.

7.2.2 Diabetes and outcomes

Diabetes has been shown in some, but not all, studies to be an independent risk factor for early and late mortality following CABG. A number of diabetes-related factors have been linked to adverse outcomes, including the following:

• More severe coronary artery disease
• Greater likelihood of left ventricular dysfunction
• Increased neointimal hyperplasia resulting in graft occlusion
• Increased risk of peri-operative complications.

7.2.3 Diabetes and peri-operative complications

Table 7.1 summarizes common post-operative complications which are more frequent in patients with diabetes. Diabetes increases the risk of superficial sternal wound infections and mediastinitis, and infections of saphenous vein or radial artery harvest sites. Saphenous vein harvest site infections may be reduced in patients with diabetes by refinements in surgical technique, including endoscopic vein harvesting. Diabetes has also been shown to be an independent risk factor for renal failure and neurological complications including stroke. The relative risk of renal failure is fivefold higher in individuals with diabetes undergoing cardiac surgery as compared to patients without. Low cardiac output syndrome is also more frequent in the presence of diabetes, suggesting that diabetes adversely affects myocardial function peri-operatively. Patients with diabetes undergoing CABG tend to stay longer on the intensive care unit post-operatively and have prolonged hospital stays, with a greater chance of re-admission, compared to patients without diabetes.

Table 7.1 Complications associated with diabetes in patients undergoing cardiac surgery

Infections	Sternal wound infections
	Mediastinitis
	Saphenous vein harvest site infection
Renal complications	Renal failure
	Requirement for dialysis
Neurological complications	Stroke
Haemodynamic complications	Low cardiac output syndrome

7.2.4 Off-pump surgery

In conventional CABG surgery, cardiopulmonary bypass is used to maintain perfusion whilst the heart is arrested for anastomosis of the bypass grafts. Recently, 'off-pump' or 'beating heart' surgery, in which anastomoses are fashioned without cardiopulmonary bypass, has become widely available. Off-pump CABG has been shown to reduce the likelihood of post-operative complications, including atrial fibrillation, renal failure, and respiratory failure, in patients with diabetes. Whether this translates in to a survival advantage for patients with diabetes undergoing off-pump CABG, however, is not yet clear.

7.2.5 Arterial revascularization

The conduits typically employed for CABG include the long saphenous veins, internal mammary artery, and radial artery. Saphenous vein conduits are prone to neointima formation, particularly in individuals with diabetes, pre-empting recurrent symptoms or graft occlusion. Arterial conduits, typically comprising internal mammary or radial arteries, are much less prone to restenosis and occlusion. In patients with diabetes undergoing CABG, the use of arterial grafts has been suggested to improve clinical outcomes including survival. The use of the left internal mammary artery for CABG has become standard practice, especially in patients with diabetes. The use of bilateral internal mammary arteries as conduits for grafting has been shown to be safe with a possible survival advantage in recent studies of patients with diabetes, but is avoided by some surgeons because of concerns over an increased risk of sternal wound infections.

7.2.6 Post-operative care

Intensive management of blood glucose levels with continuous insulin infusion has been shown to reduce morbidity and mortality in critically ill patients. A recent study of patients in the intensive care setting, the majority of whom had undergone cardiac surgery, showed a significant improvement in mortality with continuous insulin infusion. Other studies, showing reduced rates of sternal wound infection, support a policy of intensive glycaemic control in the post-operative period for patients with diabetes undergoing CABG.

7.3 Percutaneous coronary intervention

7.3.1 Percutaneous coronary intervention in diabetic patients

Patients with diabetes represent a substantial proportion of those undergoing PCI. Over the last two decades, the average age, lesion complexity, and proportion presenting with unstable coronary disease have all increased in this group. Diabetes increases the risk of procedural complications, symptom recurrence, requirements for repeat revascularization, and mortality in those undergoing PCI. Box 7.1 summarizes factors contributing to these impaired outcomes.

> **Box 7.1 Factors contributing to adverse outcomes following PCI in patients with diabetes**
>
> - Diffuse coronary artery disease
> - Increased prevalence of multivessel disease
> - Increased lesion calcification
> - Pro-thrombotic tendency
> - Resistance to antiplatelet drugs
> - Increased neointima formation
> - Increased risk of contrast-induced nephropathy.

7.3.2 Balloon angioplasty

Percutaneous Transluminal Coronary Angioplasty (PTCA) results in similar procedural success and early symptom relief in individuals with and without diabetes. However, diabetes substantially increases angiographic rates of restenosis and the requirement for repeat revascularization for recurrent symptoms. A number of factors have been implicated in the unfavourable influence of diabetes on restenosis, including the following:

- Exaggerated smooth muscle cell proliferation and hyperplasia
- Advanced glycation end products
- Inflammation
- Growth factor production in response to hyperglycaemia
- Endothelial dysfunction
- Accelerated fibrosis and altered matrix components
- Enhanced thrombogenicity
- Increased elastic recoil.

These factors are compounded by the presence of longer, more complex stenoses and greater prevalence of multivessel disease in individuals with diabetes. Restenosis culminating in occlusion of the treated vessel is a strong independent predictor of long-term mortality in patients with diabetes.

7.3.3 **Coronary stents**

Over the last decade, implantation of coronary stents has become standard practice in the vast majority of PCI procedures. Stents facilitate greater acute luminal gain, provide a mechanical scaffold to prevent elastic recoil, and reduce the effects of smooth muscle cell hyperplasia on luminal diameter. Multiple studies have shown that coronary stent deployment reduces restenosis compared to PTCA in individuals with and without diabetes. However, diabetes remains an important independent risk factor for restenosis in patients receiving coronary stents.

7.3.4 **Drug-eluting stents**

Drug-eluting stents reduce restenosis by combining the mechanical scaffolding properties of a stent with drugs which inhibit vascular smooth cell proliferation and migration. Drugs such as paclitaxel or sirolimus (and related compounds) are typically bound to the stent struts with a polymer to facilitate controlled elution of the drug in a predictable manner after deployment. Initial clinical trials showed that drug eluting stents virtually abolished restenosis in highly selected coronary lesions. Contemporary trial and registry data from patients with a wide range of lesion types suggest that drug-eluting stents reduce the risk of restenosis by up to 70%. Although the absolute risk of restenosis remains higher in patients with diabetes, the relative reduction conferred by drug-eluting stents is preserved in the presence of diabetes.

The favourable effect of drug-eluting stents on restenosis risk has facilitated the rapid expansion of PCI to encompass treatment of increasingly more diffuse and complex types of coronary disease, including multivessel disease.

7.3.5 **Antiplatelet therapy**

The pro-thrombotic tendency associated with diabetes, which is an independent risk factor for stent thrombosis, mandates appropriate anti-platelet therapy following PCI. The use of combined oral anti-platelet drugs, typically comprising aspirin and a thienopyridine (ticlopidine, clopidogrel, or prasugrel) has become standard therapy to prevent immediate and late thrombotic complications of PCI. Recent trials have shown that adequate loading of these drugs prior to the interventional procedure reduces complications. Aspirin and a thienopyridine are usually continued between 1 and 12 months following PCI, depending on the mode of presentation (stable or unstable) and type of stent (bare-metal or drug-eluting). In a recent sub-study of the Clopidogrel in Unstable angina to Reduce Recurrent Events (CURE) trial of patients with acute coronary syndromes undergoing PCI (PCI-CURE), dual antiplatelet therapy with aspirin and clopidogrel significantly reduced the risk of cardiovascular death or recurrent MI at 1 year in the subgroup with diabetes, compared with aspirin alone.

Intravenous glycoprotein IIb/IIIa inhibitors (abciximab, eptifibatide and tirofiban) have been shown in multiple trials to reduce peri-procedural complications in high-risk patients undergoing PCI. Meta-analyses of trials reporting outcomes in subgroups with diabetes demonstrate that abciximab reduced mortality by 45% at 1 year following PCI in patients with diabetes. The effect was most pronounced in insulin-treated individuals and those receiving multiple stents. However, a more recent trial suggests that adequate pre-treatment with clopidogrel (600mg at least 2 hours prior to the procedure) may negate the benefit of abciximab administration in stable patients with diabetes undergoing elective PCI. Intensive antiplatelet therapy, including intravenous glycoprotein IIb/IIIa inhibition, remains the standard of care in patients undergoing PCI for acute coronary syndromes. Although data specific to diabetes are lacking, the direct thrombin inhibitor bivalirudin, which inhibits platelets by reducing thrombin-mediated platelet activation, is emerging as an alternative to the combination of heparin and glycoprotein IIb/IIIa inhibitors during PCI.

7.3.6 **Peri-procedural care**

Contrast-induced nephropathy is common in patients undergoing PCI and portends a significant mortality and morbidity. Diabetes is an important risk factor for contrast-induced nephropathy, along with pre-existing renal disease, low cardiac output states, and the volume of contrast used. Adequate pre-hydration and the use of iso-osmolar or non-ionic contrast agents may reduce the risk of contrast-induced nephropathy in individuals with diabetes and impaired renal function undergoing PCI. Data relating to the use of *N*-acetylcysteine for renal protection are conflicting. The only study carried out exclusively in patients with diabetes did not show a significant benefit.

Management of hyperglycaemia in patients with acute coronary syndromes is discussed in Chapter 6. In the setting of elective PCI, optimal glycaemic control is associated with lower rates of target vessel revascularization in patients with type 2 diabetes. Metformin, however, is conventionally withheld from patients undergoing PCI peri-procedurally, due to the rare possibility of metformin accumulation in patients who develop renal failure precipitating lactic acidosis.

7.4 **Percutaneous coronary intervention versus CABG**

7.4.1 **Choice of revascularization strategy**

Despite recent advances in both surgical and percutaneous techniques, patients with diabetes present specific challenges to both interventional cardiologists and cardiac surgeons undertaking coronary revascularization. A number of factors may influence the decision of whether surgical or percutaneous revascularization is chosen for an individual patient. These include the number of diseased vessels (including left main coronary artery involvement), left ventricular function and the presence or absence of co-morbidities which may increase peri-procedural risk. Several randomized controlled trials have compared surgical with percutaneous revascularization in patients with diabetes and multivessel disease, although recent technological advances in both techniques limit the relevance of this evidence base to contemporary practice.

7.4.2 **CABG versus balloon angioplasty**

The Bypass Angioplasty Revascularization (BARI) trial randomized 1829 patients with multivessel disease to either balloon angioplasty or CABG. There was no difference in survival according to revascularization strategy for the trial as a whole. However, in those with diabetes (353 patients), 7-year survival was substantially higher in the CABG group than in the angioplasty group (76.4% vs 55.7%). These findings led a number of organizations to recommend that CABG should be considered the revascularization strategy of choice for patients with diabetes. Subsequent analyses of the BARI trial suggested that survival advantage conferred by CABG was limited to patients who underwent arterial revascularization using an internal mammary artery graft, and that the mortality benefit was most apparent in those experiencing a myocardial infarction during follow-up. However, in a registry of patients with diabetes who were screened for the BARI study but not entered into the randomized trial, there was no difference in survival between those receiving CABG or angioplasty. Similarly, other randomized trials in the balloon angioplasty era did not corroborate the mortality advantage conferred by CABG in the BARI trial (Table 7.2).

Table 7.2 Selected trials of angioplasty versus CABG for multivessel disease in patients with diabetes

Trial	Patients (n)	Follow-up (years)	Mortality (%)		P-value
			CABG	PCI	
BARI	353	7	23.6	44.3	<0.001
CABRI	124	4	12.5	22.6	ns
EAST	59	8	24.5	39.9	ns
BARI-registry	339	5	14.9	14.4	ns

7.4.3 **CABG versus coronary stent deployment**

At least three randomized trials comparing CABG with coronary stent deployment for multivessel disease provide mortality data for subgroups with diabetes (Table 7.3). In the Arterial Revascularization Therapies Study (ARTS), 208 patients with diabetes and multivessel disease underwent CABG or PCI with stent deployment. Mortality was not significantly different between the surgical or percutaneous approaches but freedom from clinical events was lower in the PCI group (63.4% vs 84%), almost entirely due to an increased requirement for target vessel revascularization in those undergoing PCI. The 150 patients with diabetes in the Stents or Surgery (SOS) trial had no difference in mortality according to treatment strategy. The Angina With Extremely Serious Operative Mortality Evaluation (AWESOME) randomized 454 high-risk patients requiring revascularization to CABG or PCI. A total of 144 patients had diabetes and the majority (although not all) of individuals randomized to PCI underwent stent deployment. Mortality was similar in patients with diabetes treated by CABG or PCI.

The balance of evidence, therefore, suggests that PCI with stent deployment affords comparable survival to CABG in patients with diabetes and multivessel disease, but that freedom from angina and requirement for repeat revascularization are inferior compared with CABG (Figure 7.1).

The reduced requirements for repeat revascularization following CABG may be due to the fact that bypass grafts can maintain distal coronary perfusion even if new stenoses develop in the proximal vessel. Coronary stents, being a focal treatment, cannot 'protect' against de novo lesion development in untreated coronary segments. This difference may be exaggerated by the progressive nature of atherosclerosis in individuals with diabetes.

Table 7.3 Selected trials of stents versus CABG for multi-vessel disease in patients with diabetes

Trial	Patients (n)	Follow-up (years)	Mortality (%)		P-value
			CABG	PCI	
ARTS	208	3	4.2	7.1	0.39
SoS	150	1	0.8	2.5	ns
AWESOME	144	5	34	26	0.27

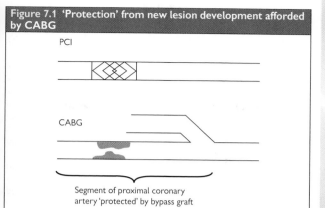

Figure 7.1 'Protection' from new lesion development afforded by CABG

PCI

CABG

Segment of proximal coronary
artery 'protected' by bypass graft

7.4.4 **CABG versus drug-eluting stents**

The advent of drug-eluting stents has substantially reduced the risk of restenosis and requirement for target vessel revascularization in patients undergoing PCI. Ongoing randomized controlled studies, including the Coronary Artery Revascularization in DIAbetes (CARDIA) and the Future REvascularization Evaluation in patients with Diabetes mellitus:Optimal Management of multivessel disease (FREEDOM) trials are testing the hypothesis that multivessel PCI with drug-eluting stents will offer comparable long-term outcomes, including freedom from angina and requirement for target vessel revascularization, to CABG in patients with diabetes.

7.5 **Conclusions**

The diffuse and rapidly progressive nature of coronary artery disease in individuals with diabetes presents significant challenges for revascularization. Despite ongoing technological refinements in surgical and percutaneous techniques, outcomes remain suboptimal compared to those without diabetes. Selection of revascularization strategy should be based on consideration of the severity and extent of coronary artery disease and the potential for complete revascularization. Current evidence suggests that contemporary PCI and CABG offer comparable survival in patients with diabetes. CABG may be preferable to bare-metal stenting in multivessel disease because of the greater freedom from angina and lower requirement for repeat revascularization. A pragmatic approach is required until the results of trials comparing drug-eluting stents with CABG are available.

Key references

Abizaid A, Costa MA, Centemero M, *et al.*, the ARTS investigators (2001). Clinical and economic impact of diabetes mellitus on percutaneous and surgical treatment of multivessel coronary disease patients. Insights from the Arterial Revascularization Therapy Study (ARTS) trial. *Circulation*, **104**: 533–8.

The BARI Investigators (2000). Seven-year outcome in the Bypass Angioplasty Revascularization Investigation (BARI) by treatment and diabetic status. *Journal of the American College of Cardiology*, **35**: 1122–9.

Berry C, Tardif JC, Bourassa MG (2007). Coronary heart disease in patients with diabetes: part II: recent advances in coronary revascularization. *Journal of the American College of Cardiology*, **49**: 643–56.

Bravata DM, Gienger AL, McDonald KM, Sundaram V, Perez MV, Varghese R, *et al.* (2007). Systematic review: the comparative effectiveness of percutaneous coronary interventions and coronary artery bypass graft surgery. *Annals of the Internal Medicine*, **147**: 703–16.

Stone KE, Chiquette E, Chilton RJ (2007). Diabetic endovascular disease: role of coronary artery revascularization. *American Journal of Cardiology*, **99**: 105B–12B.

Chapter 8

Chronic heart failure in diabetes

Miles Fisher

Key points

- Heart failure is common in people with diabetes, and diabetes is common in people with heart failure.
- Coronary heart disease and previous myocardial infarction contribute to heart failure in people with diabetes, and a diabetic cardiomyopathy is also important.
- Diastolic dysfunction is common in diabetes and may be the first sign of heart failure.
- Most of the therapies that are proved to reduce mortality in patients with heart failure are of proven benefit in diabetes. There are some particular considerations on the use of beta-blockers.
- The development of heart failure will require consideration of the most appropriate anti-diabetic drugs, and metformin and glitazones are relatively contraindicated in heart failure.

8.1 Epidemiology of heart failure in diabetes

Heart failure is the inability of the heart to pump sufficient oxygenated blood to the metabolizing tissues despite an adequate filling pressure. Chronic heart failure (CHF) can be caused by several types of cardiac dysfunction and is most commonly attributable to left ventricular systolic dysfunction (LVSD). CHF can also occur in the presence of preserved systolic function, and may be attributed to diastolic dysfunction.

Diabetes is an independent risk factor for the development of CHF, and in the Framingham study diabetes increased the risk of CHF by twofold for men and fivefold for women. There are many risk factors for the development of CHF in people with diabetes (Box 8.1), and the most important of these are hypertension and previous coronary heart disease. Around 12% of patients with diabetes in population studies have CHF, rising to 22% in patients aged more than 65 years. In people with LVSD the prevalence of diabetes ranges from 6% to 25%, increasing to 12% to 30% in patients with symptomatic CHF.

CHF carries a poor prognosis, and diabetes is an independent predictor of mortality. Diabetic patients with CHF have a higher mortality rate and rate of hospitalization compared to non-diabetic patients with CHF.

> **Box 8.1 Risk factors for the development of congestive heart failure in diabetes**
>
> - Age
> - Duration of diabetes
> - Raised HbA1c
> - Insulin use
> - Increased body mass index
> - Hypertension
> - Previous coronary heart disease
> - Retinopathy
> - Urinary albumin excretion/proteinuria
> - Nephropathy/end-stage renal disease.

8.2 Mechanisms of heart failure in diabetes

Coronary heart disease and previous myocardial infarction both contribute to chronic heart failure in diabetes. Haemochromatosis can cause both diabetes and CHF. There is also a 'diabetic cardiomyopathy' that can impair systolic emptying or diastolic filling of the left ventricle, and that contributes along with coronary heart disease to the high prevalence of CHF that is seen in people with diabetes. Several factors contribute to this cardiomyopathy, including biochemical and pathological changes in the myocardium and blood vessels (Box 8.2).

The neurendocrine responses to heart failure include activation of the renin-angiotensin-aldosterone system, activation of the sympathetic nervous system, and raised levels of serum cortisol and growth hormone. There are also increases in levels of cytokines such as TNF-alpha, IL-1, and IL-6. As exercise tolerance worsens, physical activity declines and insulin resistance increases, leading to new onset diabetes. Interestingly, new onset diabetes is more likely to occur during treatment of CHF with metoprolol than during treatment with carvedilol.

Box 8.2 Factors contributing to chronic heart failure in diabetes

Higher prevalence of conditions associated with heart failure
- Coronary heart disease
- Hypertension
- Obesity.

Other pathologies
- Diabetic cardiomyopathy
- Myocardial fibrosis
- Left ventricular hypertrophy
- Endothelial changes and dysfunction
- Diabetic cardiovascular autonomic neuropathy.

Metabolic abnormalities
- Hyperglycaemia
- Increased free fatty acids
- Insulin resistance.

8.3 Investigation of heart failure in diabetic patients

The diagnosis of chronic heart failure comprises a constellation of symptoms, signs, and the results of investigations:

- Symptoms include breathlessness, fatigue, and ankle swelling. Symptoms are used to classify heart failure in the New York Heart Association (NYHA) classification.
- Diabetic patients should be examined for the presence of clinical signs of CHF and for the complications of diabetes.
- Biochemical testing includes iron studies, HbA1c, renal function, and urine examination for microalbuminuria or proteinuria. Measurement of brain natriuretic peptide (BNP) levels, where available, is useful in people with diabetes.
- An electrocardiography (ECG) should be performed looking for previous silent myocardial infarction.
- To confirm the diagnosis of CHF cardiac dysfunction must be demonstrated. ECG will give an estimate of left ventricular ejection fraction as a measure of systolic function, diastolic dysfunction, can identify wall motion abnormalities of coronary heart disease or previous myocardial infarction, and can exclude valvular and other forms of heart disease.

8.4 **Treatment of heart failure in diabetic patients**

The approach to the treatment of CHF is similar in diabetic and non-diabetic patients, and should include the use of diuretics, angiotensin-converting enzyme inhibitors (ACE inhibitors) or angiotensin-II receptor antagonists (ARAs), and beta-blockers. CHF causes neurohormonal activation, and neurohormonal blockade with ACE inhibitors or ARBs and beta-blockers are the foundation of pharmacological therapy for CHF. Beta-blocker therapy should not be withheld in diabetic patients because of fears of hypoglycaemia.

8.4.1 **Diuretics**

Loop diuretics reduce fluid overload in patients with CHF and improve symptoms but do not appear to improve prognosis. Older studies suggested that bumetanide had less effect on glucose tolerance than furosemide, but the evidence for this in people with diabetes is minimal and either drug can be used.

In one study the aldosterone antagonist spironolactone was added to diuretics, digoxin, and ACE inhibitors in patients with LVSD and severe symptomatic CHF. Mortality was reduced by 30% overall. One quarter of the patients had diabetes and the reduction in the number of patients with diabetes was very similar. If this combination of spironolactone and ACE inhibitors is used in clinical practice there needs to be close monitoring of serum potassium and renal function in diabetic patients.

Eplerenone is a newer aldosterone antagonist that was studied following myocardial infarction in patients with LVSD and symptomatic heart failure, or diabetic patients with LVSD (one-third of the study subjects). Total mortality was reduced with eplerenone, and the benefit in patients with diabetes was similar.

8.4.2 **ACE inhibitors and ARAs**

ACE inhibitors improve the prognosis in left ventricular systolic dysfunction and CHF, and have been studied in several large multi-centre trials which have contained large numbers of subjects with diabetes. Some have published separate subgroup analysis for diabetes and have shown very similar reductions in mortality in diabetic patients with CHF. In a large meta-analysis of over 10 000 subjects in four CHF trials and three trials of post-MI ventricular dysfunction, a quarter of the patients had diabetes. ACE inhibitors reduced mortality by 14% in diabetic patients and 15% in non-diabetic subjects. Reductions were also seen in heart failure hospitalizations, and re-infarctions in patients with previous myocardial infarction with ACE inhibitors.

ARAs are an alternative to ACE inhibitors in patients who cannot tolerate ACE inhibitors because of cough, including patients with diabetes. Studies comparing ARAs and ACE inhibitors have shown conflicting results, as have studies combining ACE inhibitors and ARAs, and this combination is not routinely recommended for CHF treatment. There have been no separate published diabetes subgroup analyses for trials with ARAs, but within each study there has been no heterogeneity of effect in people with diabetes.

8.4.3 Beta-blockers

Beta-blockers have been studied in several large studies and reduce mortality in CHF. The studies included many diabetic patients, ranging from 12% to 29% of subjects, and subgroup analysis has shown similar benefits in people with diabetes and CHF. Despite this enormous evidence base, data from registers consistently show that people with diabetes and CHF are less likely to be receiving beta-blocker therapy than non-diabetic patients. This has been attributed to misguided concerns about hypoglycaemia.

The physiological response to hypoglycaemia includes activation of the autonomic nervous system. Epinephrine (adrenaline) and norepinephrine (noradrenaline) stimulate glycogen breakdown to restore blood glucose concentrations to normal. This mechanism may be antagonized by non-selective beta-blockade, prolonging the recovery from hypoglycaemia. Non-selective beta-blockade may also slightly alter the autonomic symptomatic response to hypoglycaemia. For diabetic patients with CHF these are of only minor consequence as

* Diabetic patients with CHF are often insulin resistant with poor glycaemic control, and the incidence of hypoglycaemia is low.
* The cardioselective beta-blockers bisoprolol and metoprolol can be used for the treatment of CHF.
* As described, the use of beta-blockers in diabetic patients with CHF has demonstrated beyond all doubt a reduction in total mortality and heart failure hospitalization.

All patients with diabetes, LVSD and CHF should be considered for beta-blockers in addition to ACE inhibitors, and as for non-diabetic subjects they should be used with caution in patients with bradycardia, hypotension, or chronic obstructive pulmonary disease.

8.4.4 Other drugs

Several other drugs have been studied in people with CHF including digoxin, nitrates, and hydralazine, but diabetic subgroup analysis is not available from these studies.

8.4.5 Device therapy in diabetic CHF

Cardiac resynchronization therapy pacing, also known as multi-site pacing or biventricular pacing, improves symptoms and prognosis in patients who have severe symptomatic CHF. Little diabetes data have been reported, but in two small studies diabetes subgroup analysis has shown similar improvements in morbidity and mortality in patients with and without diabetes.

There is also little specific data at present on the use of implantable cardiac defibrillators (ICDs) in diabetes. In one study no benefit was observed in a diabetes subgroup, and further research in diabetic patients is required.

8.5.5 **Surgery including cardiac transplantation**

Occasionally coronary interventions are used to improve the myocardial blood supply in patients with CHF. Cardiac transplantation is a possible treatment for patients who remain symptomatic despite optimal medical and device therapy, although the number of cardiac transplants performed has fallen since the widespread use of ACE inhibitors and beta-blockers in CHF. At first diabetes was a contraindication to transplantation, but excellent results can be obtained in selected diabetic patients. Active infection, for example, diabetic foot ulceration is a contraindication because of the immunosuppression that is required following cardiac transplantation. Large doses of steroids are used, worsening hyperglycaemia in diabetic patients and leading to new onset diabetes in many subjects who were previously non-diabetic.

8.5 **Treatment of diabetes in patients with heart failure**

The management of hyperglycaemia in diabetic patients is described in Chapter 2. Patients with CHF often have poor glycaemic control and require combinations of anti-diabetic drugs to try and improve control. There is no evidence that treatment of hyperglycaemia improves prognosis once CHF is present.

8.5.1 **Metformin**

CHF is listed as a contraindication to metformin therapy, and it is thought that heart failure increases the risk of lactic acidosis with metformin. This has now been challenged on several grounds:

- The incidence of lactic acidosis with metformin is very low.
- In case reports of lactic acidosis with metformin most have at least one other disease or illness that can result in lactic acidosis.
- A Cochrane review of 176 trials showed similar rates of lactic acidosis between metformin and other oral anti-diabetic drugs.

- Large retrospective cohort studies examining the use of metformin in patients with CHF reported either no cases of lactic acidosis, or rates of lactic acidosis that were similar to those in patients not treated with metformin.
- Large retrospective cohort studies of patients with diabetes and CHF have demonstrated that outcomes were better in patients on metformin compared to other anti-diabetic therapies, with reductions in total mortality and reduced readmissions with heart failure (Figure 8.1).

Registry studies show that despite the contraindication metformin is frequently prescribed in patients with CHF. A pragmatic approach is to use metformin in stable heart failure (NYHA classes I and II) and to withdraw metformin during episodes of cardiac decompensation, when lactate production can be increased as a result of tissue hypoxia.

8.5.2 **Glitazones**

Glitazones cause the retention of fluid through mechanisms in the distal tubules of the kidney. This may manifest itself as weight gain or ankle oedema. In a patient with early left ventricular systolic function, or diastolic dysfunction, this fluid retention can unmask heart failure, and glitazones are currently contraindicated in patients with a history of CHF.

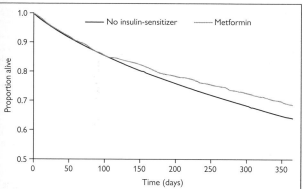

Figure 8.1 is reproduced with permission from Masoudi FA, Inzucchi SE, Wang Y, Havranek EP, Foody JM, Krumholz HM (2005). *Circulation*, **111**: 583–90.

Figure 8.1 Adjusted mortality curves for patients hospitalized with heart failure and diabetes receiving metformin at discharge and patients not treated with an insulin-sensitizing drug.

This contraindication has also been challenged on the following grounds:

- Mechanistic studies have shown improvements in myocardial insulin-stimulated glucose uptake with glitazones, with no change in left ventricular ejection fraction on echocardiography.
- In the PROactive study admissions with heart failure were increased but there was no increase in mortality or morbidity.
- Meta-analysis of randomized clinical trails demonstrated increased heart failure events but no change in cardiovascular deaths (Figure 8.2), suggesting that heart failure in patients given glitazones might not carry the same risk that is seen in CHF caused by progressive ventricular dysfunction.
- A large retrospective cohort study of patients with diabetes and CHF demonstrated a reduction in total mortality in patients prescribed glitazones, but increased readmissions with heart failure (Figure 8.3).

For the time being CHF remains a contraindication to glitazone therapy. If a patient develops fluid retention after starting a glitazone they should be investigated for CHF as described in Section 8.3. If CHF is confirmed the glitazone should be discontinued, but in the absence of left ventricular dysfunction glitazone therapy can be continued.

8.5.3 **Insulin**

In some studies insulin use has been an independent predictor of mortality in diabetic patients with CHF. It is likely that insulin use is a marker either for patients with a long duration of diabetes and extensive cardiovascular disease, or that insulin is required when other treatments are ineffective in patients with severe CHF who have neurohormonal activation that worsens insulin resistance and hyperglycaemia.

Fluid retention is a rare side effect of insulin, occurring at the start of insulin therapy in poorly controlled patients. It is caused by the direct effect of insulin on sodium and water retention in the renal tubules, and may occasionally provoke symptomatic heart failure in patients with LVSD.

8.5.4 **Other anti-diabetic drugs**

There are no contraindications to sulphonylureas in patients with CHF, but these may not control hyperglycaemia when used in isolation. There is little published experience with acarbose, or with the newer anti-diabetic drugs exenatide or the DPP-4 inhibitors.

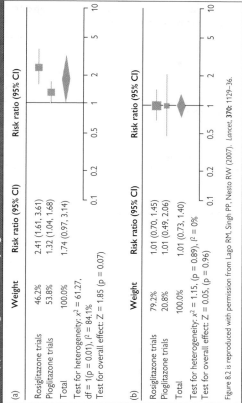

Figure 8.2 Comparison of risk of congestive heart failure (a) and cardiovascular death (b) for rosiglitazone and pioglitazone

(a)

	Weight	Risk ratio (95% CI)
Rosiglitazone trials	46.2%	2.41 (1.61, 3.61)
Pioglitazone trials	53.8%	1.32 (1.04, 1.68)
Total	100.0%	1.74 (0.97, 3.14)

Test for heterogeneity: $\chi^2 = 61.27$, df = 1 (p = 0.01), $I^2 = 84.1\%$
Test for overall effect: Z = 1.85 (p = 0.07)

(b)

	Weight	Risk ratio (95% CI)
Rosiglitazone trials	79.2%	1.01 (0.70, 1.45)
Pioglitazone trials	20.8%	1.01 (0.49, 2.06)
Total	100.0%	1.01 (0.73, 1.40)

Test for heterogeneity: $\chi^2 = 1.15$, (p = 0.89), $I^2 = 0\%$
Test for overall effect: Z = 0.05, (p = 0.96)

Figure 8.2 is reproduced with permission from Lago RM, Singh PP, Nesto RW (2007). *Lancet*, **370**: 1129–36.

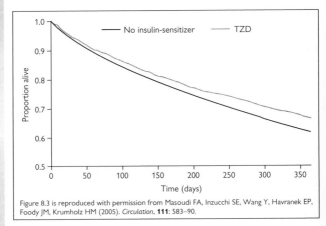

Figure 8.3 is reproduced with permission from Masoudi FA, Inzucchi SE, Wang Y, Havranek EP, Foody JM, Krumholz HM (2005). *Circulation*, **111**: 583–90.

Figure 8.3 Adjusted mortality curves for patients hospitalized with heart failure and diabetes receiving a thiazolidinedione (TZD) at dis-charge and patients not treated with an insulin-sensitizing drug.

8.6 **Conclusions**

CHF is common in patients with diabetes and can be treated in a way to similar to treating heart failure in the non-diabetic patient. The best method of treating hyperglycaemia in heart failure patients, and the risk:benefit ratios of metformin and glitazones require further research.

Key references

Bell DSH (2003). Diabetic cardiomyopathy. *Diabetes Care*, **26**: 2949–51.

Lago RM, Singh PP, Nesto RW (2007). Congestive heart failure and cardiovascular death in patients with prediabetes and type 2 diabetes given thiazolidinediones: a meta-analysis of randomised clinical trials. *Lancet*, **370**: 1129–36.

Macdonald MR, Petrie MC, McMurray JJ (2007). Diabetes, left ventricular systolic dysfunction and chronic heart failure. In M Fisher and JJ McMurray, eds. *Diabetic cardiology*, pp. 93–134, John Wiley & Sons, Ltd, Chichester, UK.

Masoudi FA, Inzucchi SE, Wang Y, Havranek EP, Foody JM, Krumholz HM (2005). Thiazolidinediones, metformin, and outcomes in older patients with diabetes and heart failure: an observational study. *Circulation*, **111**: 583–90.

Masoudi FA, Inzucchi SE (2007). Diabetes mellitus and heart failure: epidemiology, mechanisms, and pharmacotherapy. *American Journal of Cardiology*, **99**(suppl): 113B–32B.

Tahrani AA, Varughese GI, Scarpello JH, Hanna FWF (2007). Metformin, heart failure, and lactic acidosis: is metformin absolutely contraindicated? *British Medical Journal*, **335**: 508–12.

Chapter 9

Other vascular disease in diabetes

Miles Fisher

> ### Key points
>
> - Strokes are a common cause of morbidity in people with diabetes. Several secondary preventive therapies, including control of hypertension, statins, pioglitazone, and the use of anti-platelet drugs are of benefit, but aggressive management of hyperglycaemia in acute stroke carries no benefit.
> - Peripheral arterial disease is a common cause of morbidity in people with diabetes, and contributes to diabetic foot problems. Revascularization and some medical therapies may be helpful.
> - Erectile dysfunction is strongly associated with cardiovascular disease in men with diabetes, and carries a poor prognosis.
> - Renovascular disease is increased in people with diabetes, and has to be distinguished clinically from other forms of diabetic kidney disease.

9.1 Introduction

Chapters 5–8 describe the consequences of coronary heart disease in diabetes, causing stable coronary heart disease, acute coronary syndromes, and chronic heart failure, which are common causes of death in people with diabetes. Other manifestations of atherosclerotic disease are common causes of morbidity in people with diabetes, including cerebrovascular disease, peripheral vascular disease, and erectile dysfunction.

Modern studies of risk factor reduction have 'major cardiovascular disease' as one of the important endpoints, which comprises cardiovascular death, non-fatal myocardial infarction, and non-fatal stroke. Some studies will include cerebrovascular or peripheral vascular events as part of a composite endpoint (Figure 9.1). As an example,

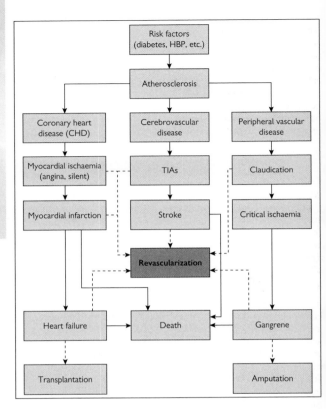

Figure 9.1 Natural history and outcomes of cardiovascular disease in different vascular beds. Some of the end points (full lines) are related to the progression of the disease, or so-called 'disease endpoints', and some are related to clinical decisions about admission or intervention (broken lines) or 'procedure endpoints'. Many composite outcomes will be a mixture of disease and procedure endpoints.

the primary endpoint in the PROactive study was a composite consisting of all-cause mortality, non-fatal myocardial infarction, stroke, major leg amputation, acute coronary syndrome, cardiac intervention including coronary artery bypass grafting or percutaneous coronary intervention, or leg revascularization.

It is well recognized that patients with atheroma in one vascular territory often have disease in other territories. In the Reduction of Atherothrombosis for Continued Health (REACH) registry of 67 888 patients with established arterial disease or high cardiovascular risk, of whom 44% had diabetes, one-sixth of the patients with coronary artery disease, cerebrovascular disease (CVD), or peripheral arterial disease (PAD) had symptomatic involvement in two or three arterial beds, confirming the diffuse nature of atherothrombosis. Many also had asymptomatic disease elsewhere. On follow-up at 1 year the event rate increased according to the number of affected vascular beds.

9.2 Strokes and Transient Ischaemic Attacks

Transient ischaemic attacks (TIAs) are classically transient neurological dysfunction lasting less than 24 hours and strokes are neurological dysfunction persisting for more than 24 hours. The risk of ischaemic stroke is increased threefold in diabetes, and encompasses a spectrum of disease from large-vessel to small-vessel occlusive disease, which may be clinically symptomatic or asymptomatic and 'silent'. There dose not appear to be any increase in haemorrhagic stroke in diabetes.

9.2.1 Pathology

In patients with diabetes there is accelerated atherothrombotic change in the large extra-cranial carotid arteries. Diabetes also increases atheroma formation in large, medium, and smaller arteries and arterioles of the cerebral circulation. In small intraparenchymal vessels there is an increase in 'microatheroma', basement membrane thickening, lipid deposition in the vessel wall, and endothelial proliferation. These pathological changes cause vessel occlusion within the microcirculation, increasing the risk of lacunar infarction in the territory of single deep-perforating arteries.

Lacunar infarction is more common in people with diabetes, and has a good prognosis for survival, but a high-risk of recurrence within the first year. Half of the patients with a lacunar stroke will have persisting disability 1 year after the initial event.

9.2.2 Management of acute stroke in diabetes

Thrombolysis with alteplase given within 3 hours of symptom onset of acute ischaemic stroke improves functional recovery. Hyperglycaemia may affect the response, and in one study admission hyperglycaemia was associated with a reduced chance of good clinical outcomes and a higher risk of intracranial haemorrhage following thrombolysis. In one observational series plasma glucose >11.2mmol/L at the time of thrombolysis was associated with a fivefold increase in the risk of intracranial haemorrhage. Some guidelines have blood glucose <2.2 or >22mmol/L as contraindications to thrombolysis in stroke.

9.2.3 Management of hyperglycaemia following stroke

Hyperglycaemia in patients with stroke carries a poor prognosis, both in diabetic patients and in patients with 'post-stroke hyperglycaemia'. This may be because of lactate accumulation and a lower survival of cells in the potentially salvageable ischaemic penumbra, and raised concentrations of glutamate, which are neurotoxic.

There are few studies that have examined the effects of intravenous insulin in stoke patients. The UK Glucose Insulin in Stroke Trial (GIST-UK) examined the effects of a glucose-insulin-potassium infusion to maintain euglycaemia following acute stroke. One in five of the subjects had type 2 diabetes. No effect was demonstrated on death or severe disability at 90 days. Study recruitment was much less than intended so the study was underpowered. Few subjects had a blood glucose concentration >10mmol/L, and the difference in blood glucose concentration between the study group and control group was only 0.6mmol/L. Further research in this area is required, and there is at least one ongoing study in the United States on the management of hyperglycaemia following acute stroke.

9.2.4 Secondary prevention of stroke in diabetic patients

Blood pressure

As described in Chapter 4 the treatment of hypertension is a powerful intervention for the primary prevention of strokes in people with diabetes, and this has also been demonstrated for secondary prevention. In the Perindopril Protection against Recurrent Stroke Study (PROGRESS) 6105 patients with a previous stroke or transient ischaemic attack were allocated to placebo, or active treatment based on perindopril, with the addition of the diuretic indapamide at the discretion of the treating physicians. Overall, there was a significant reduction in blood pressure and in recurrent fatal or non-fatal stroke. The reduction in blood pressure of 9/5mmHg was slightly greater in the diabetic subgroup of 761 patients (12%). The 38% reduction in stroke was not statistically greater than the 28% reduction in patients without diabetes. There was also a significant reduction in major coronary events and heart failure in PROGRESS. Similar results were found in the Heart Outcomes Prevention Evaluation (HOPE) study with the addition of ramipril.

Statins

Studies in patients with coronary heart disease demonstrated a reduction in strokes with statin treatment. In the Heart Protection Study (HPS), overall there was a 25% reduction with simvastatin in the first event rate for stroke, with a definite reduction in ischaemic strokes and no apparent difference in haemorrhagic strokes. Simvastatin also reduced transient ischaemic attacks and the need for carotid endarterectomy or angioplasty. Analysis of patients in HPS with prior cerebrovascular disease demonstrated no apparent reduction in the stroke rate but a significant reduction in major vascular events.

Recently, the Stroke Prevention by Aggressive Reduction in Cholesterol Levels (SPARCL) study in 4731 patients with previous stroke or TIA has demonstrated that 80mg of atorvastatin significantly reduced the primary endpoint of fatal or non-fatal stroke compared to placebo, and reduced the secondary outcome of major cardiovascular events. A total of 794 patients (17%) had diabetes, but subgroup analysis was not presented.

Hyperglycaemia

The PROactive study examined the effects of pioglitazone on recurrent vascular events in 5238 patients with type 2 diabetes and existing cardiovascular disease. A total of 984 (19%) of the patients had previous stroke disease and on follow-up there was a highly significant 47% reduction in recurrent fatal or non-fatal stroke (Figure 9.2).

Anti-platelet drugs

Anti-platelet drugs have been proven on meta-analysis to reduce recurrent vascular events, including strokes, in diabetic patients with existing vascular disease. The optimal dose of aspirin for vascular protection in people with diabetes is still uncertain.

There is very little data on other anti-platelet drugs in diabetic stroke patients. A recent study examined the role of combined clopidogrel and aspirin in patients with previous cerebrovascular disease, and 68% of the study population had diabetes. Combined therapy produced an insignificant reduction in ischaemic stroke that was offset by a higher bleeding rate.

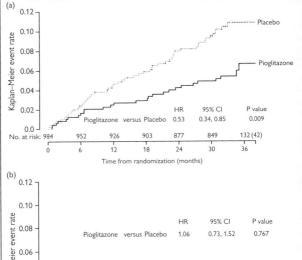

Figure 9.2 Time to stroke (fatal and non-fatal) in patients with (a) and without (b) previous stroke in the PROactive study

Figure 9.2 is reproduced with permission from Wilcox R, Bousser MG, Betteridge DJ, et al. for the PROactive Investigators. (2007). *Stroke*, **38**: 865–73.

9.3 Peripheral arterial disease

Peripheral arterial disease (PAD) is common in people with diabetes, is present in around 10% of patients at the time of diagnosis of type 2 diabetes, and will develop in up to 45% of patients on long-term follow-up. Diabetes greatly increases the risk of claudication, and the risk of non-traumatic lower limb amputation is increased between 10- and 16-fold in diabetes. Morbidity and mortality from PAD is increased in diabetes, the disease is more progressive, and the response to revascularization is less successful than in non-diabetic subjects. Risk factors for the development of PAD and for amputation are shown in Box 9.1. Diabetes tends to cause more diffuse and distal disease, and there is more vascular calcification. The clinical presentation of PAD in diabetes is shown in Table 9.1.

Box 9.1 Risk factors for PAD and amputation in diabetes

Risk factors for PAD in diabetes	Risk factors for amputation in diabetes
• Age	• Poor glycaemic control
• High HbA1c	• Age
• Raised systolic blood pressure	• Ethnicity, especially Blacks
• Low HDL cholesterol	• Smoking.
• Smoking	
• Other cardiovascular disease	
• Retinopathy	
• Sensory neuropathy.	

Table 9.1 Comparisons of peripheral arterial disease (PAD) in diabetic and non-diabetic subjects

	Diabetic	Non-diabetic
Prevalence	~ Higher	~ Lower
Age	Younger	Older
Male:Female	M = F →	M > F
Lower extremities affected	Both	Unilateral
Occlusion	Multi-segmental, distal	Single segment, proximal
Vessels involved	Tibials, peroneals	Aortic, iliac, femoral
Vessels adjacent to occlusion	Affected	Not affected
Collaterals	Affected	Not affected

9.4 **Treatment of PAD in diabetes**

Revascularization with either angioplasty or arterial bypass surgery may help to heal leg ulcers, and graft survival rate is the same as in non-diabetic subjects. The medical management of PAD in diabetes comprises an intensive multi-risk factor intervention, although the specific evidence for benefit for patients with PAD is slight, and treatment has been extrapolated from other forms of vascular disease (Table 9.2).

9.4.1 **Smoking cessation**

Smoking increases the risk of developing PAD and reduces patency rates and survival following revascularization procedures. There is little information on the effects of smoking cessation in diabetes, and the approach is similar to non-diabetic subjects with behavioural support supplemented by the use of nicotine replacement therapy or varenicline.

9.4.2 **Anti-platelet therapy**

In non-diabetic subjects anti-platelet therapy delays the progression of established PAD, but again specific data in diabetes are lacking. As for other clinical situations the optimal dose of aspirin for patients with diabetes has not been established. In the Clopidogrel versus Aspirin in Patients at Risk of Ischaemic Events (CAPRIE) study clopidogrel was more effective than aspirin in reducing myocardial infarctions and vascular deaths for patients with PAD, but data for diabetic patients with PAD were not provided.

9.4.3 **Glycaemic control**

In the UKPDS there was a trend towards a reduction in amputations and deaths from PAD in the tight control group, but this did not reach statistical significance. In the DCCT there was an insignificant reduction major lower limb complications. In the EDIC follow-up reduced peripheral arterial calcification was observed in patients who had previously been intensively treated.

Table 9.2 Multifactorial management of peripheral arterial disease (PAD) in diabetes

Risk factor	Intervention
Smoking	Smoking cessation
Thrombotic tendency	Aspirin or clopidogrel
Hyperglycaemia	Anti-diabetic drugs
Dyslipidaemia	Statins
Hypertension	Antihypertensive drugs
'At-risk foot'	Education on footcare, regular podiatry

9.4.4 **Dyslipidaemia**

In HPS patients with baseline peripheral arterial disease had a significant reduction in vascular events with simvastatin, and in patients with diabetes there was a significant reduction in a composite of peripheral vascular complications, which included any peripheral arterial surgery, peripheral angioplasty, leg amputation, or leg ulcer.

9.4.5 **Hypertension**

Hypertension is a risk factor for peripheral arterial disease, but the evidence that lowering blood pressure reduces peripheral arterial events is limited. In the HOPE study (not strictly speaking a blood pressure study) subjects with peripheral arterial disease at baseline had a highly significant reduction in the primary composite endpoint with ramipril. Overall ramipril-treated subjects had less coronary and lower extremity revascularization procedures. There should be close monitoring of renal function when ACE inhibitors are started in diabetic patients with PAD in case there is concomitant renal artery stenosis (see Section 9.6).

9.5 **Erectile dysfunction**

9.5.1 **Erectile dysfunction, diabetes, and cardiovascular disease**

The process of penile erection is a physiological neurovascular event resulting from smooth muscle relaxation, triggered and modified by neural, endocrine, and psychological components. Erectile dysfunction (ED) can be defined as the consistent or recurrent inability of a man to attain and/or maintain a penile erection sufficient for sexual performance. The association between diabetes and erectile dysfunction is well established, ED is three times more common in men with diabetes, and at least 50% of men with diabetes will suffer from ED at some time. The pathophysiology of erectile dysfunction is multifactorial and includes endothelial and smooth muscle dysfunction and autonomic neuropathy in addition to psychological and interpersonal issues.

Risk factors for the development of ED in diabetes are shown in Table 9.3. It can be seen that several risk factors for ED are also risk factors for cardiovascular disease. The link between ED and cardiovascular risk factors may be endothelial dysfunction of tissue within the corpus cavernosum. In one study ED was a marker for future cardiovascular events with a risk that was equivalent to smoking or a family history of myocardial infarction. In diabetic men ED can be associated with symptomatic coronary artery disease or silent myocardial ischaemia, and some authorities recommend screening for silent coronary disease in diabetic men who present with ED. There are also several cardiovascular medications that may be associated with an increased risk of ED (Box 9.2).

Table 9.3 Risk factors for erectile dysfunction in diabetes	
Risk factors	**Protective factors**
• Increasing age	• Increased physical activity
• Smoking	• Moderate alcohol consumption.
• Longer duration of diabetes	
• Poor metabolic control	
• Untreated hypertension	
• Neuropathy	
• Microalbuminuria	
• Macroalbuminuria	
• Retinopathy	
• Cardiovascular disease.	

Box 9.2 Drugs possibly associated with an increased risk of erectile dysfunction

Antihypertensive drugs

- Thiazide diuretcs
- Beta-blockers
- Central sympatholytics (methyldopa, clonidine)
- Spironolactone
- Calcium-channel blockers?
- ACE inhibitors?

Other cardiovascular medications

- Statins
- Fibrates
- Digoxin.

9.5.2 Treatment considerations

Oral treatments for ED are phosphodiesterase type-5 (PDE5) inhibitors, which inhibit the breakdown of cyclic GMP, and there are three available for clinical use (sildenafil, tadalafil, vardenafil). Interestingly, the effect of sildenafil on erectile function was first noticed when it was being investigated as a possible treatment for angina. PDE5 inhibitors are contraindicated in patients receiving nitrates, as the combination can cause a precipitous drop in blood pressure and coronary perfusion, in particular decreases in coronary flow rate in blood vessels with a critical coronary stenosis. Nicorandil acts as a nitric oxide donor and is also contraindicated. An expert's consensus prepared by the American Heart Association has described several relative contraindications to the use of PDE5 inhibitors in patients with cardiovascular disease (Box 9.3).

Box 9.3 Contraindications to PDE5 inhibitors

Absolute

- Nitrate therapy
- Nicorandil therapy.

Relative

- Active coronary insufficiency
- Heart failure with low blood pressure
- Patients with combination therapies involving three or four drugs for hypertension
- Patients taking anti-arrhythmic drugs with the exception of beta-blockers.

9.6 Renovascular disease

Renal artery stenosis is common in type 2 diabetes and contributes to renal impairment and hypertension. In these patients the use of ACE inhibitors or angiotensin-II receptor blockers can lead to acute renal failure, especially if renal artery stenosis affects both kidneys, or a single functioning kidney. Diabetic patients with unexplained progressive renal impairment, especially in the absence of proteinuria or retinopathy, with hypertension that is poorly controlled despite the use of multiple antihypertensive drugs, or with 'flash' pulmonary oedema should be investigated for possible renal artery stenosis. Ultrasonography is the first-line method of imaging, but a normal renal ultrasound does not exclude possible renal artery stenosis. Magnetic resonance angiography and CT angiography are the preferred non-invasive imaging modalities, and digital subtraction angiography should be reserved for patients in whom intervention is being considered, or if non-invasive imaging is inconclusive. Revascularization either by angioplasty and stenting or by direct surgical revascularization may stabilize renal function but rarely improves blood pressure management, and the place of revascularization remains uncertain.

9.7 Other vascular disease in diabetes

Atheroma affecting other vascular beds such as the gastrointestinal tract also seem to be more common in diabetes, and can be difficult to diagnose.

Key references

Berthet K, Neal BC, Chalmers JP, MacMahon SW, Bousser M-G, Colman SA, *et al.* on behalf of the PROGRESS Collaborative Group (2004). Reductions in the risks of recurrent stroke in patients with and without diabetes: the PROGRESS trial. *Blood Pressure*, **13**: 7–13.

Bhatt DL, Steg PG, Ohman EM, Hirsch AT, Ikeda Y, Mas J-L, *et al.* (2006). International prevalence, recognition, and treatment of cardiovascular risk factors in outpatients with atherothrombosis. *Journal of American Medical Association*, **295**: 180–9.

Bhasin S, Enzlin P, Coviello A, Basson R (2007). Sexual dysfunction in men and women with endocrine disorders. *Lancet*, **369**: 597–611.

Gray CS, Hildreth AJ, Sandercock PA, O'Connell JE, Johnston DE, Cartlidge NEF, *et al.*, for the GIST Trialists Collaboration (2007). Glucose-potassium-insulin infusions in the management of post-stroke hyperglycaemia: the UK Glucose Insulin in Stroke Trial (GIST-UK). *Lancet Neurology*, **6**: 397–406.

Idris I and Donnelly R (2007). Diabetes and peripheral arterial disease. In M Fisher and JJ McMurray, eds. *Diabetic cardiology*, pp. 199–222, John Wiley & Sons, Ltd, Chichester, UK.

Stroke Prevention by Aggressive Reduction in Cholesterol levels (SPARCL) Investigators (2006). High-dose atorvastatin after stroke or transient ischemic attack. *New England Journal of Medicine*, **355**: 549–59.

Wilcox R, Bousser MG, Betteridge DJ, *et al.*, for the PROactive Investigators. (2007). Effects of pioglitazone in patients with type 2 diabetes with or without previous stroke: results from PROactive (PROspective pioglitAzone Clinical Trial in macroVascular Events 04). *Stroke*, **38**: 865–73.

Chapter 10

Diabetic nephropathy

Miles Fisher

Key points

- Diabetic nephropathy develops in 40% of patients with type 1 diabetes and 30% of patients with type 2 diabetes.
- Microalbuminuria is a marker of patients who will progress to overt diabetic nephropathy, and indicates a poor cardiovascular prognosis.
- A multi-risk factor intervention for patients with type 2 diabetes and microalbuminuria reduces renal and cardiovascular outcomes.
- In type 1 diabetes the aggressive treatment of hypertension in patients with overt nephropathy with therapy based on ACE inhibitors reduces cardiovascular and renal outcomes.
- In type 2 diabetes the aggressive treatment of hypertension in patients with overt nephropathy with therapy based on ACE inhibitors or angiotensin-II receptor antagonists reduces renal outcomes, but reductions in cardiovascular events are less impressive.

10.1 Diabetic nephropathy

10.1.1 Epidemiology of diabetic nephropathy

Diabetic nephropathy is one of the principal causes of chronic kidney disease in patients starting renal replacement therapy. It is associated with a high cardiovascular mortality, and many patients with diabetic nephropathy will die from cardiovascular causes before renal function has decreased to the point where renal replacement therapy is required. The earliest stage of nephropathy is microalbuminuria, which predicts the later development of macroalbuminuria, also termed 'overt nephropathy', or 'clinical nephropathy'. Microalbuminuria is also a strong predictor of cardiovascular events in patients with type 1 and type 2 diabetes, and is included as one component in the WHO definition of the 'metabolic syndrome'.

Ten per cent of patients with type 1 diabetes will develop microalbuminuria after 7 years, and on long-term follow-up 40% will develop macroalbuminuria if untreated. In patients with type 2 diabetes a quarter will have microalbuminuria after 10 years. The prevalence of macroalbuminuria varies from 5% to 20% because of the increased cardiovascular mortality, but because of the much greater prevalence of type 2 diabetes this is still the most common type of diabetes in patients requiring renal replacement therapy.

10.1.2 **Nephropathy and cardiovascular risk**

The poor prognosis of patients with microalbuminuria may be a reflection of generalized endothelial dysfunction. Slight reductions in glomerular filtration rate also significantly increase cardiovascular risk. Further reduction in renal function leads to hypertension, left ventricular hypertrophy, accelerated coronary heart disease, and a dilated cardiomyopathy, which manifest clinically as angina, myocardial infarction, chronic heart failure, and premature death. There is also a close association between diabetic renal failure, peripheral vascular disease, foot ulcers, gangrene, and amputations.

10.2 **Microalbuminurua**

10.2.1 **Microalbuminuria and type 1 diabetes**

In patients with type 1 diabetes regression of microalbuminuria is relatively common, and regression is associated with shorter duration of diabetes, lower systolic blood pressure, tighter control of glycaemia, and lower concentrations of cholesterol and triglycerides. Once microalbuminuria is established, the aggressive treatment of glycaemia and of hypertension reduces the progression from microalbuminuria to overt nephropathy, and ACE inhibitors have effects that are partly independent of blood pressure lowering. ACE inhibitors can slow the progression of renal disease in patients with type 1 diabetes who are normotensive.

10.2.2 **ACE inhibitors, microalbuminuria, and type 2 diabetes**

Several small studies have shown beneficial effects of ACE inhibitors on microalbuminuria in patients with type 2 diabetes. In addition, trandolapril has been shown to prevent the development of microalbuminuria in patients with type 2 diabetes. The large Microalbuminuria, Cardiovascular and Renal Outcomes in the Heart Outcomes Prevention Evaluation (MICRO-HOPE) diabetes substudy from the Heart Outcomes Prevention Evaluation (HOPE study) examined the effects of ramipril on cardiovascular and renal outcomes in people who mostly had type 2 diabetes. The primary endpoint of cardiovascular death, myocardial infarction, and strokes was significantly reduced with ramipril. Renal endpoints were included in secondary outcomes, but unfortunately sampling for microalbuminuria and proteinuria was performed infrequently throughout the study. There was a significant reduction in the progression of microalbuminuria with ramipril, and a significant reduction in the development of overt nephropathy (Table 10.1).

The Diabetes, Hypertension, cardiovascular events, and Ramipril (DIABHYCAR) study examined the effects of low-dose ramipril (1.25mg) on cardiovascular and renal outcomes in patients with type 2 diabetes and raised excretion of urinary albumin. Ramipril lowered blood pressure slightly, and favoured regression from microalbuminuria to normal, but had no effect on a composite outcome of cardiovascular death, non-fatal myocardial infarction, stroke, heart failure hospitalization, or end-stage renal failure, or on any components of the endpoint.

This study suggests that low-dose ACE inhibition may reduce albumin excretion, but not cardiovascular or renal outcomes which require full-dose ACE inhibition.

10.2.3 Angiotensin-II receptor antagonists, microalbuminuria, and type 2 diabetes

Angiotensin-II receptor antagonists (ARAs) have been studied in patients with type 2 diabetes. The Irbesartan in Patients with Type 2 Diabetes and Microalbuminuria Study (IRMA-2) compared irbesartan in two doses (150mg, 300mg) with placebo in patients with hypertension and microalbuminuria. Irbesartan reduced the progression to persistent albuminuria and increased regression to normal albumin excretion. A similar, shorter study with valsartan (Microalbuminuria Reduction with Valsartan, MARVAL) showed similar benefits compared to amlodipine, indicating that some of the reduction in albumin excretion was related to blood pressure reductions and some to the specific agent. There have been a few other publications from the IRMA-2 study that have given useful information about microalbuminuria and type 2 diabetes (Box 10.1). In the IRMA-2 study mean blood pressure with 300mg irbesartan was 141/83mmHg. Some guidelines have blood pressure targets for patients with microalbuminuria that are lower than this, but the evidence for lower targets is small.

Table 10.1 Results from the MICRO-HOPE study

Cardiovascular	Renal
Reduced myocardial infarction	Reduced overt nephropathy
Reduced strokes	Reduced mean albumin:creatinine ratio
Reduced cardiovascular deaths	Reduced new microalbuminuria (not significant)
Reduced total mortality	
Reduced revascularizations	

Box 10.1 Results from the IRMA-2 study

Principal results

- In hypertensive patients with type 2 diabetes and microalbuminuria irbesartan reduced the progression to persistent albuminuria. There was a slightly greater reduction in systolic blood pressure with irbesartan compared to the placebo group.

Other cardiovascular results

- 24-Hour ambulatory blood pressure monitoring in a subpopulation of IRMA2 showed that irbesartan was renoprotective independently of beneficial effects in lowering 24-hour blood pressure.
- Irbesartan reduced markers of low-grade inflammation, including high-sensitivity C-reactive protein and fibrinogen, and attenuated the increase in interleukin-6 (IL-6). Changes in IL-6 were associated with changes in albumin excretion, and the reduction in low-grade inflammation with irbesartan may have reduced the risk of microvascular and macrovascular disease.
- One month after withdrawal of treatment, blood pressure rose in the patients who received irbesartan, but urinary albumin excretion was persistently reduced in the patients who had received irbesartan 300mg after withdrawal of therapy.

The Diabetics Exposed to Telmisartan and Enalapril (DETAIL) study compared the effects of the ARA telmisartan with the ACE inhibitor enalapril in a small group of patients with type 2 diabetes and early nephropathy. Eighty per cent had microalbuminuria, and half had a history of cardiovascular disease. The primary endpoint was the change in the glomerular filtration rate, and the effects of the two drugs were not significantly different. There was no difference in the rates of end-stage renal disease or cardiovascular events, which were secondary endpoints. Similar results were found in a smaller, shorter study which found equal reductions in blood pressure, urinary albumin excretion, and rate of decline in glomerular filtration rate comparing losartan and enalapril in hypertensive type 2 diabetic patients with early nephropathy.

Several short-term studies have examined the effects of combining ACE inhibitors and ARAs in diabetic patients with microalbuminuria. The combination leads to greater reductions in blood pressure and microalbuminuria than a single drug, but long-term studies examining the effects of the combination on the progression to overt nephropathy in diabetes, and on cardiovascular outcomes, are awaited.

10.2.4 **Other drugs**

Aliskiren is a novel renin inhibitor which blocks the renin–angiotensin system and lowers blood pressure. A short study in type 2 diabetes showed a reduction in albumin excretion in patients with type 2 diabetes and microalbuminuria, and long-term studies on the progression of nephropathy and on cardiovascular outcomes are under way.

10.2.5 **Multifactorial risk intervention for microalbuminuria**

The Steno-2 study was a comparison of targeted, intensified, multifactorial intervention with conventional treatment in a small group of patients with type 2 diabetes and microalbuminuria. Interventions in the intensive therapy group comprised of the following:

- Advice on diet, exercise, and smoking cessation
- Intensive blood glucose control with a target HbA1c below 6.5%
- The use of an ACE inhibitor irrespective of blood pressure
- Aggressive treatment of hypertension
- Statins for raised cholesterol and fibrates for raised triglycerides
- Aspirin
- Vitamin and mineral supplementation.

More patients in the intensive group reached targets for blood pressure, lipids, and HbA1c, and the blood glucose targets were the hardest to achieve. Patients receiving intensive therapy had a significantly lower risk of cardiovascular disease, nephropathy, retinopathy, and autonomic neuropathy, with a 50% reduction in events over 8 years (Figure 10.1). When specific cardiovascular events were examined the reduction in strokes was statistically significant, but the reductions in myocardial infarction and coronary interventions (PCI or CABG) did not reach individual statistical significance (Figure 10.2).

10.2.6 **Antioxidants**

In the Steno-2 study a multivitamin preparation was included as antioxidant treatment. Many large, multi-centre studies, including large numbers of patients with type 2 diabetes, have examined the possible reduction in cardiac events with antioxidant therapy, and these have been negative. A large study examining the possible benefits of aspirin and/or multivitamins in patients with type 2 diabetes is currently being run in the United Kingdom.

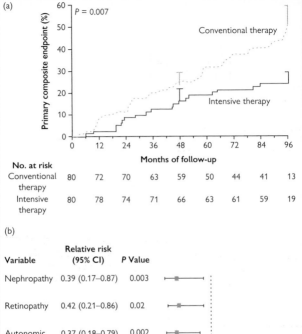

Figure 10.1 Effects of intensive multifactorial intervention in type 2 diabetes in the Steno-2 study

(a)

No. at risk

Conventional therapy	80	72	70	63	59	50	44	41	13
Intensive therapy	80	78	74	71	66	63	61	59	19

(b)

Variable	Relative risk (95% CI)	P Value
Nephropathy	0.39 (0.17–0.87)	0.003
Retinopathy	0.42 (0.21–0.86)	0.02
Autonomic neuropathy	0.37 (0.18–0.79)	0.002
Peripheral neuropathy	1.09 (0.54–2.22)	0.66

Figure 10.2 Effects of intensive multifactorial intervention in type 2 diabetes on cardiovascular events in the Steno-2 study

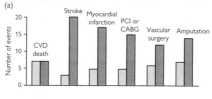

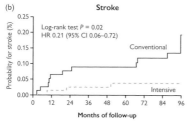

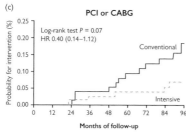

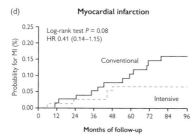

Figure 10.2 is reproduced with permission from Gaede P and Pedersen O (2004). *Diabetes*, **53**: S39–47.

10.3 **Macroalbuminuria treatments**

A small but detailed study from the Steno Hospital, Denmark, that was performed in the 1980s demonstrated that aggressive antihypertensive treatment, based on treatment with metoprolol, hydralazine, and furosemide, reduced albuminuria and the decline in glomerular filtration rate in patients with type 1 diabetes and overt nephropathy.

10.3.1 **ACE inhibitors and type 1 diabetes**

A larger, multi-centre study performed by the Collaborative Study Group compared the ACE inhibitor captopril with placebo in 409 patients with type 1 diabetes and diabetic nephropathy. Target blood pressure goals were set for all subjects. Captopril reduced the primary endpoint which was a doubling of the base-line serum creatinine concentration. There was also a significant reduction in a combined endpoint of death, dialysis, and transplantation. There were 8 deaths in the captopril group and 14 in the placebo group, but individual causes of death were not reported.

10.3.2 **Angiotensin-II receptor antagonists and type 2 diabetes**

There are several small studies showing that ACE inhibitors reduce proteinuria and the decline in glomerular filtration rate in patients with type 2 diabetes and overt nephropathy, but none of these studies was statistically powered to look at the progression to end-stage renal replacement or cardiovascular outcomes. Two large multi-centre studies were performed using the ARBs losartan and irbesartan in patients with type 2 diabetes and overt nephropathy, and there was criticism of the ethics of the study design as comparisons were made with placebo or amlodipine, and not with ACE inhibitors which were deemed to be the best treatment at the time the studies were designed.

In the Reduction of Endpoints in NIDDM with the Angiotensin-II Antagonist Losartan (RENAAL) study losartan reduced the primary endpoint which was a composite of doubling of base-line creatinine concentration, end-stage renal disease, or death. When the components of the composite were examined, losartan reduced the doubling or serum creatinine and end-stage renal disease, but had no effect on deaths. There was no effect on a secondary composite of morbidity and mortality from cardiovascular causes, although the rate of first hospitalization for heart failure was significantly lower with losartan (Figure 10.3).

There have been multiple other publications from the RENAAL study, including several that have given useful information about cardiovascular risk and nephropathy in type 2 diabetes (Box 10.2).

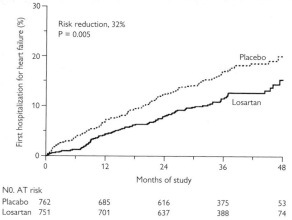

Figure 10.3 Reduction in heart failure hospitalizations with losartan in the RENAAL study

Figure 10.3 is reproduced with permission from Brenner, B.M., Cooper, M.E., de Zeeuw D, Keane WF, Mitch WE, Parving HH, *et al.*, for the RENAAL Study Investigators. (2001). *New England Journal of Medicine*, **345**: 861–9. © 2001 Massachusetts Medical Society. All rights reserved.

Box 10.2 Results from the RENAAL study

Principal results

- In patients with type 2 diabetes and overt nephropathy losartan reduced the primary outcome which was a composite of doubling of base-line creatinine, end-stage renal disease, or death.

Other important results

- Elderly patients (>65 years) had the same level of benefit and risks from treatment with losartan.
- Base-line systolic blood pressure was a stronger predictor than diastolic blood pressure of renal outcomes and death.
- Base-line total and LDL cholesterol and triglyceride levels were associated with increased risk of developing the primary composite endpoint, and were not adversely affected by losartan.
- ECG criteria of base-line left ventricular hypertrophy was associated with a significantly increased risk of cardiovascular events and the progression of kidney disease.
- Among all the base-line risk markers, albuminuria was the strongest predictor of cardiovascular outcomes, and reducing albuminuria in the first 6 months appeared to afford cardiovascular protection.

In the Irbesartan Diabetic Nephropathy Trial (IDNT) irbesartan reduced the same primary endpoint of a doubling of the base-line serum creatinine concentration, end-stage renal disease, or death compared to placebo and amlodipine, indicating that protection was independent of reductions in blood pressure. There was no significant effect on death as a component of the primary endpoint, or in a secondary cardiovascular composite end point, although the rate of hospitalization for heart failure was lower with irbesartan than with placebo.

There have been several other publications from the IDNT study that have given useful information about cardiovascular risk and diabetic nephropathy in type 2 diabetes (Box 10.3).

Box 10.3 Results from the IDNT study

Principal results

- Irbesartan was effective in protecting against the progression of nephropathy in type 2 diabetes, independently of reductions in blood pressure.

Other important results

- Further analysis of the cardiovascular composite showed a lower incidence of congestive cardiac failure with irbesartan compared with placebo, a trend towards a decrease in strokes in patients receiving amlodipine, and a significantly lower rate of myocardial infarction with amlodipine compared with placebo.
- Clinically unrecognized myocardial infarction that was detected by the development of Q waves on the electrocardiogram accounted for 14% of all non-fatal myocardial infarctions.
- The degree of albuminuria at base-line and lower serum albumin levels provided additional prognostic information about the risk of cardiovascular events in addition to traditional coronary risk factors.
- An achieved systolic blood pressure approaching 120mmHg and diastolic blood pressure of 85mmHg were associated with the best protection against cardiovascular events. A blood pressure below 120/85mmHg was associated with an increase in cardiovascular events.

10.3 Systematic reviews and meta-analysis

As mentioned above there are very few studies comparing ACE inhibitors versus Angiotensin-II receptor antagonists in patients with diabetic nephropathy. In an attempt to determine which class of drug might lead to better outcomes systematic reviews have been performed of renal and cardiovascular outcomes, and the results of these have been controversial. One systematic review concluded that there were survival benefits of ACE inhibitors for patients with diabetic nephropathy, with a reduction in all-cause mortality compared to that with placebo. Much of this evidence came from the Collaborative Study Group study of captopril in type 1 diabetes and from the MICRO-HOPE study.

By contrast, ARAs did not have any effect on all-cause mortality, and much of this data came from the IRMA-2, IDNT, and RENAAL studies. A possible biological rationale for the benefit of ACE inhibitors but not of ARAs could be the accumulation of bradykinin with ACE inhibitors (see also Chapter 4). In a similar meta-analysis which included data from LIFE, IDNT, and RENAAL studies no effect was seen on total mortality or cardiovascular morbidity and mortality.

10.4 **Other drugs to reduce cardiovascular risk**

Other than treating blood pressure with drugs that block the renin–angiotensin system there is little evidence for benefit of other interventions in people with established nephropathy. Anaemia is more common in diabetic kidney disease than other forms of kidney disease, can occur when renal function is only moderately impaired, and adversely affects the cardiovascular prognosis. There is an ongoing debate as to what is the optimal target haemoglobin for therapy with erythropoetin or analogues in renal patients, and there are several ongoing cardiovascular endpoint studies that include many patients with diabetes.

Statins have been examined in patients with renal failure, and the results have been negative. One study that examined the possible benefits of fluvastatin in patients with renal failure from multiple causes including diabetic nephropathy was negative. Another study examined the possible effects of atorvastatin in diabetic patients on haemodialysis and was also negative. The lack of a reduction in cardiovascular endpoints with statins (and angiotensin-II receptor blockers) may partly be explained by advanced nature of the atherosclerosis in these patients.

10.5 **Conclusions**

Diabetic nephropathy is associated with a high cardiovascular mortality which worsens with increasing albumin excretion and deterioration in glomerular function. Aggressive treatment of blood pressure with drugs that block the renin–angiotensin system delays the deterioration in renal function and the need for end-stage renal replacement therapy. The evidence for reductions in cardiovascular events is less impressive, and is mostly from the use of ACE inhibitors.

Key references

Brenner BM, Cooper ME, de Zeeuw D, Keane WF, Mitch WE, Parving HH, *et al.*, for the RENAAL Study Investigators (2001). Effects of losartan on renal and cardiovascular outcomes in patients with type 2 diabetes and nephropathy. *New England Journal of Medicine*, **345**: 861–9.

Heart Outcomes and Prevention Evaluation (HOPE) Study Investigators (2000). Effects of ramipril on cardiovascular and microvascular outcomes in people with diabetes mellitus: results of the HOPE study and MICRO-HOPE substudy. *Lancet*, **355**: 253–9.

Gaede P, Vedel P, Larsen N, Jensen GVH, Parving HH, Pedersen O (2003). Multifactorial intervention and cardiovascular disease in patients with type 2 diabetes. *New England Journal of Medicine*, **348**: 383–93.

Gross JL, de Azevedo MJ, Silveiro SP, Canani LH, Caramore ML, Zelmanovitz T (2005). Diabetic nephropathy; diagnosis, prevention, and treatment. *Diabetes Care*, **28**: 178–88.

Lewis EJ, Hunsicker LG, Bain RP, Rohde RD (1993). The effect of angiontensin-converting-enzyme inhibition on diabetic nephropathy. The Collaborative Study Group. *New England Journal of Medicine*, **329**: 1456–62.

Lewis EJ, Hunsicker LG, Clarke WR, Berl T, Pohl MA, Lewis JB, *et al.*, for the Collaborative Study Group (2001). Renoprotective effect of the angiotensin-receptor antagonist irbesartan in patients with nephropathy due to type 2 diabetes. *New England Journal of Medicine,* **345**: 851–60.

Parving H-H, Lehnert H, Brochner-Mortensen J, Goms R, Andersen S, Arner P, *et al.*, for the Irbesartan in Patients with Type 2 Diabetes and Microalbuminuria Study Group (2001). The effect of irbesartan on the development of diabetic nephropathy in patients with type 2 diabetes. *New England Journal of Medicine*, **345**: 870–8.

Chapter 11

Diabetic autonomic neuropathy and sudden death in diabetes

Miles Fisher

Key points

- Symptomatic diabetic autonomic neuropathy is uncommon in type 1 diabetes, but may cause postural hypotension and may limit exercise tolerance.
- Symptomatic autonomic neuropathy carries a poor prognosis and sudden cardio-respiratory arrest is described.
- Asymptomatic abnormalities of cardiac autonomic function are common in patients with type 1 diabetes and type 2 diabetes.
- A syndrome of 'dead in bed' is described in type 1 diabetes in patients with long-standing diabetes, which may be caused by nocturnal hypoglycaemia in patients with abnormal autonomic function provoking serious arrhythmias.

11.1 Clinical description of diabetic autonomic neuropathy

Diabetes is the most common cause of autonomic neuropathy in developed countries. Symptomatic autonomic neuropathy is a late complication of diabetes. It is typically seen in patients who also have a distal sensorimotor polyneuropathy. The autonomic nervous system controls the electrical and contractile activity of the heart through an interaction of sympathetic and parasympathetic fibres. 'Cardiac autonomic neuropathy' indicates dysfunction of the autonomic nerves to and from the heart, and 'cardiovascular autonomic neuropathy' includes damage to the fibres enervating the heart and blood vessels, resulting in abnormalities of heart rate and blood pressure control. Patients with symptomatic autonomic neuropathy have a poor prognosis and the cause of death is often cardio-respiratory arrest or sudden death.

11.1.1 Epidemiology and aetiology

Testing for autonomic neuropathy is not done routinely so there is little information about the epidemiology of diabetic autonomic neuropathy. Studies have tended to be cross-sectional rather than prospective, have included short follow-up periods, and different methods of assessment have been used. Asymptomatic abnormalities are common when testing autonomic cardiovascular reflexes in diabetes, and may be found in 40% of patients. Risk factors for cardiovascular autonomic neuropathy are described in Box 11.1. Although hyperglycaemia and duration of diabetes have major roles, insulin resistance and hyperinsulinaemia also play a part. There is also a strong association with diabetic nephropathy.

Box 11.1 Risk factors for diabetic cardiovascular autonomic neuropathy

- Age
- Duration of diabetes
- Poor glycaemic control
- Hypertension
- Dyslipidaemia
- Obesity
- Lack of physical fitness
- Smoking
- Diabetic nephropathy
- Retinopathy
- Distal symmetrical polyneuropathy ('peripheral neuropathy').

11.2 Symptomatic cardiovascular autonomic neuropathy

11.2.1 Resting tachycardia and palpitations

The resting heart rate is higher in diabetic populations compared with non-diabetic populations, reflecting early parasympathetic neuropathy, although this is still usually within the normal range of <100 beats per minute. As the parasympathetic vagal neuropathy worsens a true resting tachycardia (>100 beats per minute) develops because of unopposed sympathetic stimulation. This may be noticed by the patient and may occasionally give a sensation of palpitations. With more profound sympathetic neuropathy the heart rate lowers again, and in severe neuropathy the heart rate is fixed and does not respond to exercise or other stimuli.

11.2.2 **Postural hypotension**

Postural or 'orthostatic' hypotension is a fall in blood pressure in response to a change in posture from lying to standing. It occurs because of an efferent sympathetic vasomotor denervation with reduced vasoconstriction of splanchnic and other vascular beds. It can cause symptoms of weakness, dizziness, faintness, visual upset, pre-syncope, or syncope. By contrast, some diabetic patients may have profound drops in systolic blood pressure on standing, which are completely asymptomatic.

Postural hypotension can be difficult to treat, and simple measures such as fluid repletion and salt supplementation or wearing support stockings are often ineffective. Fludrocortisone may relieve symptoms by expanding plasma volume, and a sympathomimetic agent such as midodrine can be added if symptoms persist (Figure 11.1).

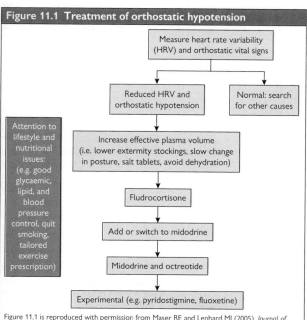

Figure 11.1 Treatment of orthostatic hypotension

Measure heart rate variability (HRV) and orthostatic vital signs

↓

Reduced HRV and orthostatic hypotension → Normal: search for other causes

Attention to lifestyle and nutritional issues: (e.g. good glycaemic, lipid, and blood pressure control, quit smoking, tailored exercise prescription)

Increase effective plasma volume (i.e. lower extermity stockings, slow change in posture, salt tablets, avoid dehydration)

↓

Fludrocortisone

↓

Add or switch to midodrine

↓

Midodrine and octreotide

↓

Experimental (e.g. pyridostigmine, fluoxetine)

Figure 11.1 is reproduced with permission from Maser RE and Lenhard MJ (2005). *Journal of Clinical Endocrinology and Metabolism*, **90**: 5896–903.

11.2.3 **Reduced exercise capacity**

The physiological response to exercise includes reduction in parasympathetic neural tone and activation of the sympathetic nervous system, including direct effects via sympathetic stimulation and indirect effects secondary to the release of epinephrine (adrenaline) from the adrenal medulla. This enhances cardiac output and increases blood flow to skeletal muscle. These mechanisms can be affected by autonomic neuropathy, reducing the heart and blood pressure responses to exercise, with a lesser increase in cardiac output, and a reduced exercise tolerance which is noticed by the patients as early fatigue. Reduced ejection fraction, systolic dysfunction, and decreased diastolic filling also limit exercise tolerance.

11.2.4 **Silent myocardial ischaemia**

Strictly speaking, this is the absence of a symptom related to neuropathy of the afferent pain fibres which are carried from the heart in the vagus nerve. Silent myocardial ischaemia is more common in people with diabetes, and is partly explained by a cardiovascular autonomic neuropathy (see also Chapter 5). As pain is a symptom that leads the patient to attend a doctor and undergo further investigation, the presence of silent or atypical ischaemia delays investigation and may partly explain the increase in sudden fatalities from acute myocardial infarction in diabetes.

11.3 **Assessment of autonomic function**

Simple assessment of autonomic function can be performed using a battery of non-invasive cardiovascular reflex tests (Box 11.2). These involve the measurement of changes in heart rate and blood pressure in response to a range of physiological stimuli that reflect changes in parasympathetic and sympathetic outflow to the heart and blood vessels. They can be performed in the consulting room or at the bedside using a blood pressure device and an ECG machine to record the R-R interval. Previously it was felt that the heart rate tests assessed parasympathetic function and blood pressure test sympathetic function, and that parasympathetic abnormalities preceded abnormalities of sympathetic function, but using more sophisticated tests it is clear that many of these tests assess both branches of the autonomic nervous system and that damage to the sympathetic activity probably occurs in parallel to parasympathetic damage.

> ### Box 11.2 Tests of cardiovascular autonomic function in diabetes
>
> **Cardiovascular autonomic reflex tests**
> - Heart rate response to deep breathing
> - Heart rate response to standing
> - Heart rate response to the Valsalva manoeuvre
> - Systolic blood pressure response to standing
> - Diastolic blood pressure response to sustained handgrip.
>
> **Other cardiovascular tests**
> - 24-Hour heart rate variation
> - Power spectral analysis
> - Spontaneous baroreflex sensitivity
> - Cardiac radionuclide imaging.

11.3.1 Heart rate response to deep breathing

The heart rate response to deep breathing mostly assesses parasympathetic function. Several different techniques of deep breathing are described, but paced deep breathing, for example, at six breaths per minute, is probably most reliable. Similarly, several different measures of heart rate variation during deep breathing have been described.

11.3.2 Heart rate response to standing

On initial standing, withdrawal of parasympathetic tone increases the heart rate. In response to subsequent blood pressure changes a baroreflex mediated reflex activates sympathetic nerves. In normal subjects there is a rapid increase in heart rate on standing, maximal at around the 15th beat with a relative slowing that is maximal around the 30th beat. The ratio of the 30th:15th beat should normally be >1.0. In the presence of autonomic neuropathy the increase in heart rate is slower, and the ratio will be <1.0. Refinements of the test include taking measures from 20 to 40 beats and 5 to 25 beats, and measuring the ratio of the longest to shortest R–R interval.

11.3.3 Heart rate response to the Valsalva manoeuvre

The heart rate response to the Valsalva manoeuvre is influenced by both parasympathetic and sympathetic activity. In normal subjects the response during the strain is vasoconstriction and an increase in heart rate, and there is an overshoot of blood pressure and a slowing of the heart rate following the release of the strain. The patient forcibly exhales against a fixed resistance for 15 seconds and the Valsalva ratio is the ratio of the longest R–R interval after the manoeuvre to the shortest R–R interval during the manoeuvre. In autonomic neuropathy the increase in heart rate during the strain is reduced, so the ratio is reduced.

11.3.4 Systolic blood pressure response to standing

A change from lying to standing activates afferent receptors from baroreceptors which increases efferent sympathetic impulses and causes an increase in peripheral vascular resistance and an increase in heart rate, with little change in blood pressure. In patients with autonomic neuropathy baroreflex compensation is impaired so blood pressure falls. A fall in systolic blood pressure of >30mmHg is abnormal.

11.3.5 Diastolic blood pressure response to sustained handgrip

Sustained isometric contraction is tested using a handgrip dynometer which assesses a reflex arc involving both afferent and efferent fibres from muscles. The efferent fibres innervate the heart and muscle, increasing heart rate, blood pressure, and cardiac output. A normal response is an increase in diastolic blood pressure of >15mmHg, and a rise of <10mmHg is abnormal.

11.3.6 Other tests of cardiac function

There are several other newer tests of the heart that require more sophisticated equipment (Box 11.2). A reduction in 24-hour heart rate variability is thought to be more sensitive than the standard reflex tests and may be able to detect cardiac autonomic neuropathy earlier. The sympathetic innervation of the heart can be visualized and quantified using the myocardial uptake of the radionuclide meta-iodobenzylguanidine (MIBG), and in cardiovascular autonomic neuropathy there is a decrease in uptake.

11.4 Prognosis of diabetic autonomic neuropathy

In patients with diabetic cardiovascular autonomic neuropathy there is an increase in total mortality and sudden death, and in patients with symptomatic autonomic neuropathy mortality may be over 50% on 5- to 10-year follow-up. A meta-analysis has shown a greater risk for studies that defined neuropathy with the presence of two or more abnormalities compared with studies that used one measure (Figure 11.2).

Cardio-respiratory arrest is well described in patients with symptomatic diabetic autonomic neuropathy, and there are several other possible explanations for the increased mortality associated with diabetic autonomic neuropathy (Box 11.3).

Figure 11.2 Relative risks for studies of cardiovascular autonomic neuropathy (CAN) and mortality

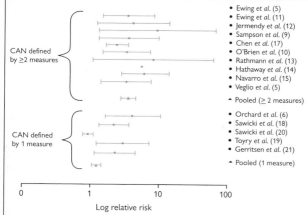

CAN defined by ≥2 measures
- Ewing et al. (5)
- Ewing et al. (11)
- Jermendy et al. (12)
- Sampson et al. (9)
- Chen et al. (17)
- O'Brien et al. (10)
- Rathmann et al. (13)
- Hathaway et al. (14)
- Navarro et al. (15)
- Veglio et al. (5)
- ▲ Pooled (≥ 2 measures)

CAN defined by 1 measure
- Orchard et al. (6)
- Sawicki et al. (18)
- Sawicki et al. (20)
- Toyry et al. (19)
- Gerritsen et al. (21)
- ▲ Pooled (1 measure)

Log relative risk

Figure 11.2 is reproduced with permission from Maser RE, Mitchell BD, Vinik AI, Freeman R (2003). *Diabetes Care*, **26**: 1895–901.

Box 11.3 Possible causes of death in autonomic neuropathy

- Concomitant cardiac or renal disease
- Absent or altered perception of myocardial ischaemia
- Deficient response to stress such as surgery, infection, or anaesthesia
- Increased predisposition to arrhythmia because of QT interval prolongation
- Changes in cardiac sympathetic/parasympathetic balance.

11.4.1 QT interval prolongation

Many studies have shown increases in the QT interval in patients with diabetic autonomic neuropathy. In non-diabetic subjects increases in the QT interval are associated with an increased risk of sudden death, so this is one possible linking factor between diabetic autonomic neuropathy and sudden death.

11.5 Sudden death in diabetes

Sudden and unexpected death of a young person is a rare but well described occurrence in non-diabetic subjects. It was suggested that the frequency of sudden death in type 1 diabetes increased following the introduction of the use of human insulin into clinical practice, and that this increase was caused by hypoglycaemia. This was subsequently named the 'dead in bed syndrome'. Estimates of sudden death in type 1 diabetes suggest that the risk is double that of the non-diabetic population, but a clear link with hypoglycaemia has not yet been established.

11.5.1 Dead in bed syndrome

The British Diabetic Association, (now Diabetes UK) collected a detailed series of sudden, unexpected deaths of young people with type 1 diabetes, referred by pathologists, diabetes physicians, and relatives of people with diabetes. Fifty-three cases were referred and many were excluded because a definite cause of such as suicide, self-poisoning, ketoacidosis, or hypoglycaemic brain damage death was identified.

Twenty-two patients were classified as 'dead in bed'. They tended to be on multiple insulin injections and free of diabetic complications. All died outside hospital, 19 were sleeping alone at the time of death, and 15 died during the night. 20 patients were found in an undisturbed bed. Few had any of the known risk factors for confirmed death from hypoglycaemia (Box 11.4). Fourteen patients had a history of severe nocturnal hypoglycaemia, and the scenario was consistent with an episode of severe or protracted nocturnal hypoglycaemia having precipitated sudden death. As there was no neuropathological evidence of hypoglycaemic brain damage a sudden cardiac or respiratory arrest was implicated. Post-mortem biochemical testing for possible hypoglycaemia was not performed, and in any case it is notoriously unreliable with many false positives and false negatives for hypoglycaemia.

Sudden, unexpected death in patients with type 1 diabetes has now been described in several countries, and some risk factors are suggested (Box 11.4).

11.5.2 Possible mechanisms of sudden death

In the general population the most frequent cause of sudden death is a cardiac arrhythmia, mostly related to coronary heart disease. Some of the increase in sudden death in diabetes will be the consequence of premature coronary heart disease, but this was excluded in the cases described. In some patients hypoglycaemic convulsions may contribute, but again this was circumstantially excluded by the fact that most subjects were found in an undisturbed bed.

The two additional possible contributions to sudden death in diabetes are autonomic neuropathy and hypoglycaemia. A plausible explanation is a combination of the changes in the QT interval which accompany nocturnal hypoglycaemia but fails to waken the patients unless symptoms are intense, occurring on a background of early autonomic neuropathy, provoking fatal arrhythmia (Box 11.5).

Box 11.4 Risk factors for death from hypoglycaemia and risk factors for 'dead in bed syndrome' in patients with type 1 diabetes

Risk factors for death from hypoglycaemia
- Alcoholism and/or inebriation
- Psychiatric illness or personality disorder
- Self-neglect or malnutrition
- Fecklessness/resistance to education
- Diabetes secondary to pancreatic disease
- Hypopituitarism following pituitary ablation.

Risk factors for 'dead in bed syndrome'
- Previous nocturnal hypoglycaemia
- Living/sleeping alone
- Intensive insulin therapy
- Multiple injections of insulin
- Alcohol ingestion.

Box 11.5 Possible mechanisms of sudden death in type 1 diabetes

Autonomic neuropathy
- Prolongation of the QT interval
- Reduced heart rate variability
- Diminished baroceptor sensitivity.

Hypoglycaemia
- Activation of the autonomic nervous system
- Increased plasma epinephrine (adrenaline) and lowering of serum potassium
- Prolongation of the QT interval
- Autonomic imbalance during hypoglycaemia.

11.6 **Treatment of diabetic autonomic neuropathy**

Intensive glycaemia control can slow the development and progression of autonomic neuropathy in type 1 and type 2 diabetes. Some drugs have been shown to improve measures of autonomic dysfunction, including the beta-blocker metoprolol, the ACE inhibitor quinapril, and the angiotensin-II receptor antagonist losartan, but the long-term effects on mortality are not known.

There is a strong association between autonomic neuropathy and microalbuminuria, and recently a paradigm for treating diabetic patients with autonomic dysfunction has been suggested (Figure 11.3). Before this is accepted into routine practice, however, studies are required to see if these pharmacological interventions consistently improve autonomic function, and whether this translates into better exercise tolerance or reduced mortality; this approach should be considered experimental at present.

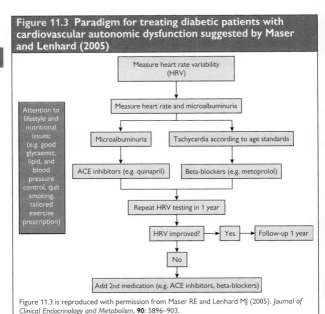

Figure 11.3 Paradigm for treating diabetic patients with cardiovascular autonomic dysfunction suggested by Maser and Lenhard (2005)

Measure heart rate variability (HRV)

Attention to lifestyle and nutritional issues: (e.g. good glycaemic, lipid, and blood pressure control, quit smoking, tailored exercise prescription)

Measure heart rate and microalbuminuria

Microalbuminuria — Tachycardia according to age standards

ACE inhibitors (e.g. quinapril) — Beta-blockers (e.g. metoprolol)

Repeat HRV testing in 1 year

HRV improved? — Yes → Follow-up 1 year

No

Add 2nd medication (e.g. ACE inhibitors, beta-blockers)

Figure 11.3 is reproduced with permission from Maser RE and Lenhard MJ (2005). *Journal of Clinical Endocrinology and Metabolism*, **90**: 5896–903.

11.7 **Conclusions**

Abnormalities of cardiovascular autonomic neuropathy are common on testing of cardiovascular reflexes, but symptomatic autonomic neuropathy is uncommon, and carries a poor prognosis. Large multi-centre studies of possible pharmacological interventions are required to reduce the high cardiovascular mortality associated with symptomatic autonomic neuropathy.

Key references

Fisher M and Heller SR (2007). Mortality, cardiovascular morbidity and possible effects of hypoglycaemia on diabetic complications. In BM Frier and M Fisher, eds. *Hypoglycaemia in clinical diabetes*, pp. 265–83, John Wiley & Sons, Ltd, Chichester, UK.

Maser RE and Lenhard MJ (2005). Cardiovascular autonomic neuropathy due to diabetes mellitus: clinical manifestations, consequences, and treatment. *Journal of Clinical Endocrinology and Metabolism*, **90**: 5896–903.

Maser RE, Mitchell BD, Vinik AI, Freeman R (2003). The association between cardiovascular autonomic neuropathy and mortality in individuals with diabetes. *Diabetes Care*, **26**: 1895–901.

Tatersall RB and Gill GV (1991). Unexplained deaths of type 1 diabetic patients. *Diabetic Medicine*, **8**: 49–58.

Vinik AI, Maser RE, Mitchell BD, Freeman R (2003). Diabetic autonomic neuropathy. *Diabetes Care*, **26**: 1553–79.

Vinik AI and Ziegler D (2007). Diabetic cardiovascular autonomic neuropathy. *Circulation*, **115**: 387–97.

Chapter 12

Health economic aspects of treating cardiovascular disease in diabetes

Ailsa Brown, Joyce Craig, and Ken Paterson

Key points

- Scarce resources in health-care systems mean that choices have to be made on how resources are spent.
- Economic evaluations are increasingly used in health-care decision making to provide an indication of the cost-effectiveness of different treatment options.
- The cost-effectiveness ratios of treatments for glycaemic control, lipid-lowering, blood pressure control, and management of established cardiovascular disease are generally within a range that is considered cost-effective in the United Kingdom.

12.1 Economic evaluation of health care

Health economic assessments are increasingly being used in health-care decision making, as evidenced by the use of economic analyses by organizations such as the National Institute for Health and Clinical Excellence (NICE) and the Scottish Medicines Consortium (SMC). Their use relates to a basic problem in economics, resolving the issues of scarcity and choice. Scarcity of resources exists in health-care systems worldwide and means that there will never be sufficient funds to meet all the competing demands for health care. Choices therefore have to be made about how to spend resources in order to meet the objectives of the health-care system. Economic evaluation techniques can provide a systematic way of considering solutions to the problem of scarcity and choice by allowing comparison of the costs and consequences of two (or more) alternative health-care interventions.

12.1.1 **The incremental cost-effectiveness ratio**

It is clear from the preceding chapters that there are many different treatments available to treat cardiovascular disease in people with diabetes; each treatment will give rise to a specific pattern of costs and effects. For example, in trying to manage a patient's weight, clinicians could use lifestyle interventions or drug therapy. If drug therapy provided greater benefits but at an increased cost compared to lifestyle modification, then economic evaluation can provide a marker to help the decision maker judge whether the additional benefits justify the additional costs. In comparing treatment options in an economic evaluation, the convention is to calculate the additional benefit provided by the more effective treatment and then present the findings in terms of 'cost per additional unit of benefit', for example, 'cost per additional life year gained'. This ratio of incremental cost to incremental benefit is known as the incremental cost-effectiveness ratio (ICER).

12.1.2 **Quality-adjusted life year**

Many treatments offer a range of effects such as improved quality of life and prolonged survival. Cost-effectiveness analysis using an outcome measure such as 'cost per additional life year gained' struggles to take account of both dimensions of benefit. Another commonly used measure of benefit seen in economic evaluations is the quality-adjusted life year (QALY). The QALY adjusts length of life for quality of life by assigning a value between zero and one (where zero represents death and one represents perfect health) for each year of life. Figure 12.1 illustrates the concept of a QALY.

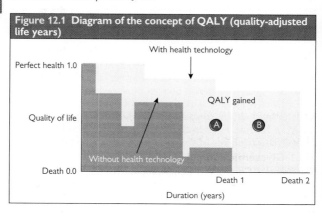

Figure 12.1 Diagram of the concept of QALY (quality-adjusted life years)

Without the new health technology the individuals' quality of life, measured on the y axis, would deteriorate over time until they die ('death 1'). However, with the technology the individuals' quality of life is maintained at a higher level and they survive some years longer than with the original treatment ('death 2'). Area A represents the quality of life gain with the new treatment while area B corresponds to the survival gain with the treatment. Added together, they represent the total QALY gain associated with the new treatment. QALYs thus have the advantage of capturing gains in quality of life and survival in a single measure.

12.1.3 **Health economic models**

Data from a variety of sources (clinical trials, disease registries, epidemiological studies) are often combined to develop a health economic model of the disease and the effects of interventions. Costs of the new treatment can be offset by savings from adverse events avoided as well as the from clinical benefits of improved quality of life and survival. Benefits are often extrapolated beyond the data that are available (e.g. from a 2-year clinical trial to 10 years or even the patient's lifetime) and this, along with other aspects of the modelling, requires assumptions to be made. The impact of varying these assumptions, either individually or in combination, is tested in sensitivity analyses, giving a range of ICERs from best to worst case scenarios. This reveals which assumptions are key to the cost per QALY and may allow key assumptions to be underpinned by additional data.

To assess if the treatment is cost-effective, the resulting 'cost per QALY' ratio can be compared either to similar ratios for other interventions already adopted by the health service or to the decision maker's stated willingness to pay for an additional QALY. In the United Kingdom, NICE uses a rule of thumb that a cost per QALY of less than £20 000 is generally considered to be cost-effective.

The remainder of this chapter will discuss the findings of selected published economic evaluations on the principal treatment options in this population.

12.2 **Cost-effectiveness of improved glycaemic control**

12.2.1 **Glycaemic control in type 1 diabetes**

The Diabetes Control and Complications Trial (DCCT) is discussed in Chapter 2. Alongside this clinical trial, an economic evaluation was conducted. An economic model was developed to estimate the lifetime benefits and costs of intensive insulin therapy compared to conventional therapy. Data from other clinical trials and epidemiologic studies were used to model the probabilities of longer-term complications such as blindness, end-stage renal disease (ESRD), and amputations. The model was structured around the occurrence of events such as retinopathy, nephropathy, neuropathy, and death, though because DCCT did not demonstrate a difference in macrovascular complications, macrovascular disease states were not explicitly modelled. Intensive insulin therapy was more expensive than conventional care but resulted in fewer deaths and fewer expensive-to-treat microvascular complications such as blindness, amputation, and ESRD. The resulting cost per QALY gained was $19 987 (at 1994 US dollars), leading the authors to conclude that intensive insulin therapy is a cost-effective treatment option.

12.2.2 **Glycaemic control in type 2 diabetes**

UKPDS has also been discussed in Chapter 2. An economic evaluation was an integral part of this trial. As with DCCT, information from the trial was combined with other data to estimate the lifetime costs and effects of the various treatment options considered in the trial. Microvascular and macrovascular complications were included in the model. The cost per QALY gained from intensive treatment compared to conventional treatment was £6028. The use of metformin in overweight patients was found to be both cheaper and more effective than conventional treatment. These results suggest that the intensive blood glucose control strategies studied in UKPDS should be considered cost-effective compared to other accepted uses of health-care funds in the United Kingdom. The results rely on those of UKPDS and it should be noted that as UKPDS was conducted between 1977 and 1991, standards of conventional care are likely to have improved. This may affect the relative costs and effects of intensified glycaemic control compared to current conventional care.

12.2.3 **Cost-effectiveness of thiazolidinediones in type 2 diabetes**

Several economic evaluations have recently investigated the cost-effectiveness of adding a thiazolidinedione to existing treatments. A study based on the PROactive trial estimated that the cost per QALY gained from adding pioglitazone to existing treatment in patients at a high risk of cardiovascular events was £4060. This analysis was based on the Centre for Outcomes Research (CORE) diabetes model, which has been used in several economic evaluations in diabetes. In the model, any improvement in baseline HbA_{1c} as a result of a novel treatment is assumed to be sustained. There is the possibility that, while an improvement in HbA_{1c} may be observed over the short-to-medium term, this improvement may be eroded in the longer term, which could alter (increase) the stated ICER.

The model also assumes that the benefits of lowered HbA_{1c} are the same, irrespective of which treatment has led to the lowering.

Recent controversy around data on rosiglitazone has cast doubts on this assumption, and the reliability of published assessments of the cost-effectiveness of rosiglitazone is therefore questionable.

12.3 Cost-effectiveness of blood pressure control in type 2 diabetes

In addition to investigating the cost-effectiveness of glycaemic interventions, tight blood pressure control was also investigated as part of UKPDS. A policy of tight blood pressure control was associated with a cost per QALY gained of £369 compared to a less tight blood pressure control target, reflecting the low costs of the drugs used in blood pressure management in UKPDS. This very low ICER would not apply to use of newer, more expensive blood pressure lowering drugs.

12.4 Cost-effectiveness of statin therapy for primary and secondary prevention of CVD in people with diabetes

A recent health technology assessment compared statin therapy to no treatment for people with diabetes. The analysis assumed that statins achieved a similar relative risk reduction from baseline CVD event rates for people with diabetes and those without diabetes. Because people with diabetes are at higher absolute risk of CVD events the absolute benefit, measured by events avoided, is greater for this group.

For those with diabetes and a history of CVD, the incremental cost per QALY was below £9000 for all age groups. For primary CVD prevention in people with diabetes, the incremental cost per QALY was under £17 500 for all those aged less than 75 years, rising to £27 600 for men aged 85 years.

The analysis used a weighted average annual cost of statins of £317. Simvastatin has since become available as a generic product and its annual cost has fallen from the £297 used in the model to under £50. The sensitivity analyses in the assessment showed that a 40% reduction in price was associated with a 36% reduction in the cost per QALY. The cost per QALY with generic simvastatin will be even lower than this as the ICER is clearly very sensitive to drug cost. These analyses suggest that treatment with statins is cost-effective for primary and secondary prevention of CVD in all people with diabetes.

This conclusion is supported by a more recent analysis of the cost-effectiveness of giving 40mg simvastatin daily to almost 6000 people with diabetes, 90% of whom had type 2 diabetes. These were included in a randomized controlled trial of 20 536 people. The economic evaluation combined the clinical trial data and UK hospital admission event costs, using an annual cost for simvastatin of £63.50. The results showed that lifetime use of the statin was cost-saving for people with type 2 diabetes (i.e. the cost of the simvastatin was less than the savings from the hospitalization events avoided).

12.5 **Cost-effective strategies to manage people with diabetes and established CVD**

Established CVD includes patients with ST-segment elevation myocardial infarction (MI) and non-ST-segment elevation acute coronary syndromes (ACS). The main management strategies are medical therapy or early primary angioplasty. Choices within the latter include primary angioplasty with bare metal stents or drug-eluting stents, or coronary artery bypass surgery. This section reviews the evidence on the cost-effectiveness of these strategies.

12.5.1 **Cost-effective management of people with diabetes and ST-segment elevation myocardial infarction**

A recent study compared the cost-effectiveness of primary angioplasty to medical management using thrombolytic drugs to achieve reperfusion after an ST-segment elevation MI.

The clinical data were from a meta-analysis of 22 randomized controlled trials and costs were from UK NHS sources. The meta-analysis reported greater clinical benefits from angioplasty compared to thrombolysis for all clinical outcomes but the benefits were very dependent on the time delay to undertake the angioplasty.

A model was developed assuming a time delay of 54 minutes for angioplasty, the mean time reported in the clinical studies. The incremental cost per QALY for primary angioplasty compared to medical management was £9241, with a 90% probability that primary angioplasty would be cost-effective at a threshold of £20 000. If the time delay to perform angioplasty was 90 minutes, the incremental cost per QALY increased to £64 750.

There is no analysis of the relative effect of angioplasty across patient subgroups, including patients with diabetes. It is thus not clear at present whether the relative benefits and impact of time delays are the same for people with diabetes as for those without diabetes.

12.5.2 Cost-effective management of people with diabetes and non-ST-segment elevation ACS

No robust evidence comparing the cost-effectiveness of strategies to manage patients with diabetes and ACS has been found. However, several health technology assessments on the wider patient group with ACS suggest evidence for the following:

- Angioplasty can be cost-effective compared to medical therapy for patients with chronic stable angina (£1743 per patient free of angina – no cost per QALY estimate).
- It is cost-effective to include intravenous glycoprotein IIb/IIIa antagonists as initial medical management (ICER £5738 per QALY).
- Angioplasty with stents, compared with coronary artery bypass grafting, for patients with multi-vessel disease, and particularly for those with diabetes, is not cost-effective (ICER £62 000 per QALY at 5 years follow-up).

12.6 Conclusions

This brief review of the cost-effectiveness of selected treatments for people with diabetes supports prescribing statins for primary prevention and angioplasty rather than medical management for initial treatment of acute coronary syndromes. Strategies of intensive blood glucose control and tight blood pressure control are also cost-effective uses of health-care resources. New interventions will have to demonstrate clinical benefits to justify any increased cost relative to existing proven managements.

Key references

Bravo Vergel Y, Palmer S, Asseburg C, Fenwick E, de Belder M, Abrams KR, et al. (2007). Is primary angioplasty cost effective in the UK? Results of a comprehensive decision analysis. *Heart*, **93**: 1238–43.

Clarke PM, Gray AM, Briggs A, Stevens RJ, Mathews DR, Holman RR on behalf of the UK Prospective Diabetes Study. (2005.) Cost-utility analysis of intensive blood glucose and tight blood pressure control in type 2 diabetes (UKPDS 72). *Diabetologia*, **48**: 868–77.

Diabetes Control and Complications Trial Research Group (1996). Lifetime benefits and costs of intensive therapy as practiced in the diabetes control and complications trial. *Journal of American Medical Association*, **276**: 1409–15.

Drummond MF, Sculpher MJ, Torrance GW, O'Brien BJ, Stoddart GL (2005). *Methods for the economic evaluation of health care programmes*. 3rd Edition. Oxford University Press, Oxford.

Heart Protection Study Collaborative Group. (2006). Lifetime cost-effectiveness of simvastatin in a range of risk groups and age groups derived from a randomised trial of 20 536 people. *British Medical Journal*, **333**: **1145**(2 December), doi:10.1136/bmj.38993.731725.BE.

Hill R, Bagust A, Bakhai A, Dickson R, Dundar Y, Haycox A, *et al.* (2004). Coronary artery stents: a rapid systematic review and economic evaluation. *Health Technology Assessment*, **8**(35): 1–242.

Robinson M, Palmer S, Sculpher M, Philip Z, Ginnelly L, Bowens A, *et al.* (2005). Cost-effectiveness of alternative strategies for the initial medical management of non-ST elevation acute coronary syndrome: systematic review and decision-analytical modelling. *Health Technology Assessment*, **9**(27): 1–158.

Sculpher MJ, Petticrew M, Kelland KL, Elliott RA, Holdright DR, Buxton MJ (1998) Resource allocation for chronic stable angina: a systematic review of effectiveness, costs and cost-effectiveness of alternative interventions *Health Technology Assessment*, **2**(10): 1–176.

Valentine WJ, Bottomley JM, Palmer AJ, Brandle M, Foos V, Williams R, *et al.* on behalf of the PROactive Study Group. (2007). Proactive 06: cost-effectiveness of pioglitazone in type 2 diabetes in the UK. *Diabetic Medicine*, **24**: 982–1002.

Ward S, Lloyd Jones M, Pandor A, Holmes M, Ara R, Ryan A, *et al.* (2007). A systematic review and economic evaluation of statins for the prevention of coronary events. *Health Technology Assessment*, **11**(14): 1–160.

Index